# Nurse-Led Clinics

In recent years there has been a huge growth in nurse-led clinics within hospital outpatient departments, general practitioner surgeries and walk-in centres. The government has endorsed the use of such clinics as a way for the public to access specialist healthcare and treatment more quickly and also as an effective way to manage chronic ill health.

However, there is a lack of uniform structure in educational preparation for nurses interested in taking up nurse-led practice and a dearth of literature offering practical guidance. *Nurse-Led Clinics: Practice Issues* provides a much-needed overview of this expanding arena for nursing and includes case studies from practitioners running nurse-led clinics. Topics covered include:

- setting up a clinic
- public protection issues
- nurse education
- managing medicines
- effectiveness and evaluation

As nurse-led clinics expand, notably into areas traditionally seen as the domain of medicine, the need to maintain a measurably effective service becomes a priority. This text allows the reader to explore key practice issues which directly affect the quality of service provided. It will be an invaluable handbook for nurses directly involved in running clinics, for those responsible for the provision of nurse-led services and for nurse educators.

**Richard Hatchett** trained as a Registered General Nurse specialising in cardiac and intensive care nursing before taking up his current post as Principal Lecturer in the Faculty of Health and Social Care at London South Bank University. His interest in nurse-led clinics stems from Masters level work at City University, London. He has published widely and is co-editor of *Cardiac Nursing: A Comprehensive Guide*.

# Nurse-Led Clinics

## Practice Issues

## Edited by Richard Hatchett

Routledge
Taylor & Francis Group

NEW YORK AND LONDON

First published 2003
by Routledge
2 Park Square, Milton Park, Abingdon, Oxon, OX14 4RN

Simultaneously published in the USA and Canada
by Routledge
270 Madison Ave, New York, NY 10016

Transferred to Digital Printing 2005

*Routledge is an imprint of the Taylor & Francis Group*

Typeset in Times by Wearset Ltd, Boldon, Tyne and Wear
Printed and bound in Great Britain by TJI Digital, Padstow, Cornwall

*British Library Cataloguing in Publication Data*
A catalogue record for this book is available from the British Library

*Library of Congress Cataloging in Publication Data*
Nurse-led clinics : practical issues / edited by Richard Hatchett.
    p. ; cm.
Includes bibliographical references and index.
    1. Nurse practitioners–Great Britain. 2. Clinics–Great Britain.
    [DNLM: 1. Nurse Clinicians–organization & administration–Great
Britain. 2. Nurse Clinicians–standards–Great Britain. 3. Nursing
Process–Great Britain. 4. Professional Practice–Great Britain. WY128
N9727 2003] I. Hatchett, Richard.
    RT82.8.N847 2003
    362.1'0941–dc21
                                                              2003008309

ISBN 0-415-28311-6 (hbk)
ISBN 0-415-28312-4 (pbk)

# Contents

# Illustrations

## Figures

## Boxes

# Contributors

**Richard Hatchett**, principal lecturer, Faculty of Health and Social Care, London South Bank University. Interests in cardiac nursing in primary and secondary care, the implementation of the nurse-led clinic, the history of ministerial workforce policy and planning.

**Lynda Filer**, lecturer in applied biological sciences, St Bartholomew School of Nursing and Midwifery, City University, London. Interests in pharmacology in clinical practice, nurse prescribing and medicines management.

**Emma Pennery**, formerly senior clinical nurse specialist/honorary lecturer and research fellow, Royal Marsden Hospital and Institute of Cancer Research, London. Interests in breast cancer management, breast care nursing, advanced nursing practice issues and the needs of women with breast cancer following treatment.

**Catriona Sutherland**, clinical nurse specialist in contraception and women's health, Paxton Green Group Practice, London. Interests in sexual health, notably with young people, nurse education/development.

**Shelley Mehigan**, clinical nurse specialist, family planning, The Garden Clinic, Sexual Health Service, Slough Primary Care Trust (PCT) and Redwood House Surgery, Maidenhead. Member of the fpa clinical advisory committee. Interests in nurse prescribing, contraceptive implant fitting and removal, nurse education/development.

**Alison Pottle**, cardiology nurse consultant, Royal Brompton and Harefield NHS Trust, based at Harefield Hospital. Interests in low density lipoprotein (LDL) apheresis, care of the patient pre- and post-percutaneous transluminal coronary angioplasty (PTCA), notably psychological support; chest pain clinics and expanding nursing roles.

**Sara Da Costa**, nurse consultant in diabetes, Worthing and Southlands Hospitals NHS Trust and Visiting fellow, University of Brighton. Interests in leadership, mentoring, motivational interviewing in patient focussed consultations and new role implementation.

# Preface – San Francisco 1992

In August of 1992 I took a month's break from my job as a cardiac charge nurse and travelled across the United States on a delta pass. A delta pass was a flat rate open ticket which meant that within a specified time period you could virtually live on Delta Airline's domestic flights, flying from city to city and seeing the States. I travelled from New York up to Boston, down to Washington, over to Nashville and Chicago and eventually came down on the West Coast in San Francisco. Throughout the journey, I called into various hospitals, having completed my US exams in Britain, and with the need for more familiar surroundings in such a large country. In San Francisco I was due to visit the ambulatory AIDS clinic, at the San Francisco General Hospital, a short bus ride from the salubrious surroundings of the YMCA where I was staying. I remember it well, because I left my wallet on the counter at the hostel at breakfast, and had to hurry back off the bus and up the street to retrieve it before reaching the hospital.

The ambulatory clinic was in fact an outpatients department. It was a bustling, restless and people filled area, with a small desk at one end, doors down one side and as I remember, a corridor somewhere on the other side. The staff were welcoming but busy, and I waited for a while at the reception desk surveying the scene. By that stage AIDS had wreaked havoc on San Francisco and the room was heaving and filled with a slight air of agitation. I remember clearly in the midst of all this, a fragile, skeletal young man with the back of his head resting against the wall, eyes closed. The whole gamut of the disease seemed to be present in that room.

Eventually I was able to watch what I would come to know as the advanced nurse practitioner in one of the several clinical rooms. These were large and white, and appeared remarkably quiet compared to what lay outside their doors. Each nurse chatted engagingly and caringly to the patients, mostly men of varying ages and carried out a systematic clinical assessment of their illness. They seemed to know the personal details, which come from frequent visits, and chatted about all sorts of social titbits as they examined. Glands in various parts of the body were palpated, mouths were inspected and pulse oximetry was used to detect reducing oxygen haemoglobin saturations, an early sign of pneumocystis carinii pneumonia. A small bank of doctors saw patients who the nurses felt needed a medical consultation and who reviewed test results and X-rays.

This was my first experience of what I came to know, less than a decade later, as the nurse-led clinic. Nursing was adapted and expanding its skills to meet the needs of an overwhelming problem and where patients need good, prompt healthcare. It remained an excellent example of meeting the needs of a chronic illness, which we now believe works so well with the nurse-led clinic, where health can be monitored and assessed, with the ultimate aim of optimising the health status. With their need for competency based professional development and good evaluation, nurse-led clinics have grown enormously in the United Kingdom in the last decade.

When considering this and nurses expanding their practice, it's not unusual to see debates presented which argue that nurses can or cannot replace doctors. This I believe misses the fundamental point of the nurse-led clinic, advanced nurse practitioner, nurse consultant and other nursing roles. Nursing is not in competition with medicine, it's a case of considering who can provide the most appropriate service to the patient. If we continually compare ourselves to medicine, it suggests once again a hierarchy with medicine at the top, and a smug satisfaction that we could have performed many of their roles all along. In addition this reflects back to an era when nursing attempted to emulate the professional trait gains of medicine, and were inevitably reduced to that derogatory term a 'semi profession'.

In preparing this book I have had the pleasure of working with some of the healthcare professionals whose writing I have enjoyed and who have inspired me over the years. I also thank all of the small and knowledgable teams involved in this overall project. This book is dedicated to all the nurses who have been brave enough to grasp the need for adaptation to meet changing healthcare needs. May your remuneration be as high as your enthusiasm.

Richard Hatchett
London 2003

# Acknowledgements

Sincere thanks for the support and advice of the following in the writing of this book

| | |
|---|---|
| Thomas Aird | Satwant Singh |
| Lynda Filer | Ben Halligan |
| Mary Saunders | Jackie Knight |
| Andrea Bellot | Paul Warburton |
| Wendy Johnson | Karen Rawlings Anderson |
| Professor Carol Cox | Emma Martin |
| Shelley Mehigan | Catriona Sutherland |
| Catriona Minnock | Elaine Coady |
| Richard Lewis | Michelle Stanton |
| Hilary Hollis | Barbara Stilwell |
| Emma Pennery | Lee Thorogood |
| Gay Foxwell | Fiona Smart |
| Brian Boag | Alun Roebuck |
| Sara Da Costa | Pene Cook |
| Professor Dinah Gould | Judy Scotter |

Special thanks to Katrina Maclaine, Professor Celia Davies, Kim Manley CBE and Edwina Wellham, Karen Bowler and the team at Routledge.

## Chapter 1

# The emergence of the modern nurse-led clinic

*Richard Hatchett*

The term 'nurse-led clinic' emerged predominately within the nursing literature in the 1980s. Although historically, nurses had been running clinics of some sort before this time, there was a clear growth in a large variety of nursing disciplines of this form of healthcare provision. In addition, the clinics have coincided with an expansion of practice, which has encroached into areas normally reserved for medicine. This has included detailed physiological assessment, together with the manipulation and prescribing of medications. The rise of the nurse-led clinic has notably accelerated in the 1990s. A review of the Catalogue of International Nursing and Allied Healthcare Literature (CINAHL) database back to 1982, and utilising the term 'nurse-led clinic' reveals 41 papers, but only one prior to 1995. The British Nursing Index provides 18 papers in the seven years to 2002, while the Royal College of Nursing (RCN) Journals Database offers 11 papers from 1985 to 1996. Only three appear to occur before 1994. From this literature a useful and broad definition of the modern nurse-led clinic emerges (see Box 1.1).

This introductory chapter explores the concept of the nurse-led clinic and the areas where it has emerged. Key elements in the changing face of healthcare are presented, which are suggested as influencing the development of this form of healthcare provision. The issues in Box 1.1 generally refer to patients who have been previously diagnosed by a doctor. Here, the value of the nurse-led clinic fits into an era of an ageing population, and one which lives with chronic, rather than curable, ill health. In line with this, the 2001 census revealed that in the last 50 years the UK population has aged considerably. The proportion of those less than 16 years has now decreased from 24 per cent to 20 per cent, while those over 60 years has increased from 16 per cent to 21 per cent.

Notably, in 1951 there were 0.2 million people aged over 85 years, while the figure in 2001 was 1.1 million. This figure represents a five-fold increase (Office for National Statistics 2002). The diabetic, cardiac or respiratory patient, together with those with dermatological or rheumatology problems, may not need to see a doctor each time a deterioration in their

---

**Box 1.1    Broad definition of a nurse-led clinic**

A clinic where the nurse has his or her own patient case load. This involves an increase in the autonomy of the nursing role, with the ability to admit and discharge patients from the clinic, or to refer on to other more appropriate healthcare colleagues. This power to refer to others is often highly variable between clinics, but can include referrals to professionals allied to medicine, such as dieticians, physiotherapists, chiropodists and social work teams, through to medical teams or consultants.

An educative role – explaining the illness to the patient and carers. This includes the significance of symptoms, differentiating between those of concern that require further treatment or adjustment of medication and those that may be from alternative causes. The issues of health education and promotion fall into this category.

Psychological support – this does not appear in all of the literature focussing on nurse-led clinics, but listening to the patient's concerns, fears and perceived improvements in health is clearly an important role.

Monitoring the patient's condition – this is an area which has developed rapidly in recent years. This involves the skills of history taking and physical assessment, considering the significance of assessment and ordering further investigations. This will also involve referring on to more appropriate colleagues or initiating treatments. The emergence of Patient Group Directions (PGDs)* and nurse prescribing has meant that manipulating medications is an increasing role of the nurse-led clinic.

---

condition occurs or for ongoing assessment. The aim of the nurse-led clinic is to monitor the condition and to maintain the patient in their optimal state of health. Increasingly, this has meant a move towards empowering the patient to identify the signs of deterioration themselves, and to take appropriate action. Such action may include the use of more easily accessible specialist advice through the nurse-led clinic, a 'drop in service', or via a telephone helpline. It is pointless altering the hierarchical power boundaries between patient and service providers, if there is no readily accessible service to respond promptly to what the patient discovers.

---

*PGDs (formerly known as group protocols) emerged from the first Crown Report published in 1989 (DOH 1989). They are specific protocols created by a multidisciplinary team. This includes medical and pharmacy colleagues, and those professions likely to contribute to care under the protocol. PGDs allow a specific drug to be administered without utilising a practitioner with full prescribing rights, and are initiated when certain criteria are met (DOH 1998). As part of the review on the prescribing, supply and administration of medicines, group protocols were further explored in 1997. This review led again by Dr June Crown was the first part of the second Crown Report (DOH 1999a), in which clear criteria were written for establishing group protocols (DOH 1998). The heath service circular published in 2000 (DOH 2000a) entitled Patient Group Directions, enabled PGDs to finally come into practice.

This issue of empowerment is an important component of the nurse-led clinic. In evaluating the worth of the service, it has to be considered whether the aim is to redistribute work amongst healthcare professionals, and make accessibility to those services easier for the patient, or whether there is an aim to enable the patient to deal more effectively themselves with a variety of healthcare problems. The measurement of such empowerment needs to be off set against the frequency with which the patient comes into contact with the clinic. Such frequent contact could be seen as the factor which prevents deterioration, as opposed to an increased patient awareness of their own condition and the significance of symptoms.

Many nurse-led clinics are found either in General Practice in the community, or in the outpatients department of the hospital setting (Hatchett 2000). In the latter, the nurse tends to be specialised within one area. These can be in a large variety of quite specific but varied areas. This can include back pain management (Wallis 2000), peritoneal dialysis (Denning 2000), intermittent claudication (Binnie et al. 1999), leg ulcer management (Vowden 1997), intractable childhood constipation (Muir and Burnett 1999) and pre-admission clinics (Alderman 1997; Newton 1996; Ryan, P. 2000). The majority of this literature exploring nurse-led clinics tends to be found within the popular nursing press and often extends to only a few pages. Such papers tend to be highly positive regarding the clinics, but are generally descriptive and lack the deeper analysis, which provides insight into how and why the clinic has formed. Two important issues are how the nurse demonstrates, maintains and further develops competence in often expanding areas of practice and how the worth of the clinic is demonstrated. Professional competence is a recurring theme within this text, because of its link to both public protection and to ensuring the clinic is a valued contribution to managing healthcare, and not a second rate service emerging due to over worked medical colleagues.

In the late 1990s and early twenty-first century a new form of nurse-led clinic emerged which went beyond the boundaries of the diagnosed patient. In contrast to the clinics above, these were the services that dealt with undifferentiated, undiagnosed patients. These were basically those with a new health concern, who walked in off the street. Such services were seen with the emergence of the National Health Service (NHS) walk-in centres, 40 of which developed in the first few years of their launch in 2000, 12 alone in London. These were quite unique, and the nurses who undertook such services need praise for their bravery in initiating such ground breaking work. The centres occurred in a variety of settings, sometimes in hospital grounds, in high streets and even at an airport. They were nurse-led, although general practitioner (GP) services were available for a limited time period at some, and they were open for extended times, although not for 24 hours.

The service provided treatment for a large variety of usually self-limiting conditions such as minor wounds and burns, muscle and joint injuries, headaches, high temperature, minor infections including urinary tract, ear and nose, eye care such as conjunctivitis, emergency contraception, family planning and pregnancy testing. In increasing healthcare access, they were aimed at groups who found accessing primary care difficult, as well as the working public whose jobs often clashed with the usual general practice hours. They also aimed to relieve the overcrowding of accident and emergency departments of essentially non-emergency conditions.

An important addition has been the *NHS (Primary Care) Act* of 1997 (DOH 1997). This offered the opportunity for innovations in the delivery of primary care services. This was notably by creating more flexible ways of offering primary healthcare and inevitably meant an opportunity to set up services which were nurse-led. A series of personal medical services (PMS) pilot schemes were launched in April 1998, following finalisation in December of the previous year. Some started later than the April date, due to the shortage of time to recruit staff, create protocols and in some cases find premises (Moore 1999). Only two of the initial nine nurse-led pilot sites commenced on 1 April 1998 (Lewis 2001). A second wave of 106 projects was launched in October 1999, with a second series of 80 projects from April 2000. The third series in two parts, began in April 2001, with a total of 1,100 pilot schemes. A fourth series, again in two parts, was launched in 2002 (DOH 2002).

One of the main initiatives of the PMS pilots which were nurse-led, was to provide healthcare access to those who were regarded as living on the margins of society. This included refugees, the homeless and those with challenging behaviour, particularly if continually moved on by the police, and which made accessing healthcare difficult (Gardner 1998). A small number of the pilot schemes aimed to provide comprehensive primary care services predominately by a nurse or nursing team supported, rather than led, by GPs. Baraniak (2001) described the philosophy of her nurse-led general practice as allowing the patient to be seen by the most appropriate person to help them with their problem. This is determined by the nurse, who is the first point of contact for the patient. He/she assesses the problem, treats if skilled to do so, initiates tests or further investigations, and if appropriate refers the patient to another professional. Choice is offered to the patient regarding who they wish to see (Baraniak 2001). However, for a variety of logistical reasons, such as the failure to recruit a general practitioner or gain adequate patient numbers, some nurse-led pilot schemes floundered (Moore 1999).

Lewis (2001) provided a valuable review of the first nine PMS sites that were nurse-led. Two of the nine were run by nurses acting as independent contractors (Baraniak and Gardner 2001). Five of the pilots were managed by community NHS Trusts, and the remaining two were managed by existing general practitioner practices. The term nurse-led can be viewed as a continuum of practice ranging from the nurse having delegated authority to make decisions regarding patient care at one end of the spectrum, to being responsible for all care provided. The latter includes clinical assessment, treatment and management of patients undifferentiated by need (Baraniak and Gardner 2001). There is also however, an implicit non-clinical element, through managerial leadership. The nurse will be the team leader in much the same way that an independent contractor GP is seen as the leader. The notion did appear to cause some confusion and tension in the first wave of PMS sites and may have diminished in later sites. This was because it was never explicitly explored within the team, and therefore cut across traditional power relations between doctors and nurses. Lewis argues that this was one of the reasons behind a shift in terminology from 'nurse-led' to 'team-led'. This terminological shift represented a more fundamental clarification in practice of the values that should underpin the model, as well as a more practical equilibrium in terms of interprofessional power within a team (Richard Lewis: personal correspondence 2003).

Nurse-led primary care reflects a model of service where the nurses have a higher profile in providing care for patients, based on their own assessment of the patient's needs. Such decisions are based on the nurse's level of skill and ability, and their interpretation of the scope of practice. Decision-making is supported by practice protocols or guidelines, or by parameters set by the employer(s). For practice nurses, this employer would normally be the GP (Baraniak and Gardner 2001). Nurse-led primary care and further innovations such as Baraniak and Gardner working as independent contractors, may assist practice nurses in encouraging innovations away from possible restriction through direct employment by GPs.

Baraniak and Gardner (2001), as well as Lewis' work (2001), reviewed PMS sites that were nurse-led, but importantly provided a valuable analytical framework for all nurse-led clinics. The issues that have hindered the services are included in Box 1.2.

The issue of interprofessional relationships, notably between doctors and nurses in the nurse-led PMS sites, has been of interest. Primarily, the sites have aimed to offer the patient the most appropriate healthcare professional to meet their needs. In many cases this may not be a healthcare professional at all, but perhaps a counsellor or marriage guidance service. This is often because patients with non-medical problems, do not know where else to go for help. The philosophy is one of a changed set of relationships between clinicians in the primary care team and those between the team and their patient (Lewis 2001). This does suggest 'nurse-led' as a term is misleading, but is about equality of opportunity, mutual respect among team members and a focus on the appropriate needs of the patient. Within the concept of

---

**Box 1.2    Issues that have hindered the development of PMS nurse-led pilots, with relevance to the development of the nurse-led clinic (adapted from Baraniak and Gardner (2001) and Lewis (2001))**

A lack of nationally recognised qualifications for nurses taking on extended nursing roles. This has notably been the lack of regulation of the use of the term 'advanced nurse practitioner'. Any nurse has been able to call themselves a Nurse Practitioner and run a nurse-led clinic. The Nursing and Midwifery Council (NMC) subsequently began moves in 2003 to protect, via registration and required competencies, roles within the domain of specialist and advanced nursing practice (NMC 2003). Many had previously argued for a clear set of competencies, a specific registration to protect the public, as well as exploring the plethora of other legal issues (Maclaine 1998; RCN 2002; Walsh 2000), but the NMC had been slow to protect the title. The Royal College of Nursing produced a definition and competencies to clarify the situation, together with suggested standards for educational preparation (RCN 2002).

Prescribing rights. These are developing, but it has been a slow process for nursing.

The absence of authority outside of the hospital setting for nurses to sign sick certificates and paperwork relating to welfare benefits.

A lack of recognition of the nurse being able to certify death, even though they, rather than the doctor, may have seen the patient many times during terminal illness. At the present time it is illegal for nurses to certify death.

Securing referral rights to secondary care and other agencies. In Lewis' work, nurses were understanding of hospital doctors and consultants not wishing to receive referrals from anyone other than a doctor, because of the aforementioned lack of recognised standards and competencies to underpin the role of the nurse practitioner. Medical staff have little way of knowing the competence of the nurse who is referring a patient. Only two of the nine initial nurse-led PMS pilot sites had secured formal referral rights with NHS hospital trusts (Lewis 2001). Lewis clarifies this further by reinforcing that while only two of the nine sites in his study had agreed formal referral rights, others had negotiated informal rights with some specialists. In this context, a significant shift in traditional practice had been achieved, although it underlines the veto ability of many doctors over changes to interprofessional relationships (Richard Lewis: personal correspondence 2003).

---

the nurse-led clinic, success will always focus on being a team player and the interprofessional relationships with other colleagues.

In many of the PMS nurse-led pilots, Lewis believed, the dynamics were consistent with the philosophy, but in some that power issues prevailed. Here, GPs retained the decision on which clinician would see which patient. For two nurse leads this retaining of dominant power led to their departure within two years of their pilot's inception. Such issues were compounded by the legal fact that patients must be registered with a doctor, and he or she has the power to sign almost all prescriptions. It is also of interest that it appeared that while nurses offered services to those perhaps termed on the margins of society, medical resistance seemed muted. It appeared stronger in Lewis' work, when nurses tried to offer services to more mainstream populations.

One of the interesting occurrences within the nurse-led PMS sites was the fact that they have run the risk of creating a two-tier service. Those who traditionally had difficulty accessing primary care, such as the homeless, refugees and travelling people may have been moved on from traditional general medical services (GMS) practice to the nurse-led services, because they had been developed to meet their needs. This may let neighbouring practices 'off the hook' in relation to these patients (Lewis 2001). It may also fly in the face of an equitable NHS, with the possibility of the disadvantaged being offered nurse-led care while the rest receive GP-led services.

The important issue within this chapter is the need for practitioners in nurse-led clinics and nurse-led services to be competent in their skills. The issue of an unprotected title of nurse practitioner within the profession has not been a simple argument, and points for and against this will be discussed in Chapter 2. Baraniak and Gardner (2001) called for more formal and recognised structures to support them during their service development. The Royal College of Nursing had offered constant encouragement, but tangible support such as packages for indemnity insurance for those who have developed as independent nurse contractors in primary care, was not forthcoming. Such formal support is needed as we move somewhat rapidly into new philosophies of managing patients, and practise advanced skills as never before, supported by the push of government policy. Literature continues to emerge regarding PMS sites, with another useful report being that of Roe *et al.* (2001).

## Government support for nurse-led clinics

The Labour government was clearly a supporter of nurse-led services of which nurse-led clinics form a significant part. This move is probably supported by a variety of rationale; including offering greater access for the public to healthcare, reducing doctors' working hours, recognising the skilled abilities of the nursing profession and making a more efficient use of healthcare resources. The government's nursing strategy '*Making A Difference*' (DOH 1999b: 63) had highlighted the provision of nurse-led services to 'provide health information, self help advice and minor treatments'. In addition, the Crown Committee (DOH 1998) allowed nurses to adjust prescribed medication under specific protocols, which encouraged nurse-led practice and eased the way for nurse-led clinics.

By March 2000 Prime Minister Tony Blair was challenging the NHS to use an increased average funding of 6.1 per cent per year over the following four years, to meet changes encompassed in five challenges. The third of these asked the professions to 'strip out unnecessary demarcations, introduce more flexible training and working practices, and ensure that doctors do not use time dealing with patients who could be treated safely by other healthcare staff' (Blair 2000). Such demarcations he regarded as 'outdated' for a modern NHS. Nurses at their Royal College of Nursing congress were promised a government 'to liberate nurses.... Equality between professions, that is what I want to see. Not nurses versus doctors. But nurses and doctors working together. Each contributing their unique skills to a single care system' stated secretary of state for health, Alan Milburn (Milburn 2000). Subsequently, Milburn's nursing roles identified at RCN congress became chief nursing officer, Sarah Mullally's key roles for nurses (Box 1.3).

Within specific documents the role of nurse-led clinics was recognised. *The National Service Framework for Coronary Heart Disease* is an example (DOH 2000b: 48). This called for heart failure clinics which 'could be successfully led by nurse practitioners or doctors'. Such support had even led medical staff to complain that certain nurse-led PMS pilot schemes were funded to a greater degree than other more traditional services (Ryan, C. 2000).

## The pathway to the modern nurse-led clinic

The alteration in the division of labour between healthcare professions must in part be attributed to the changing attitude to the concepts of the professions. The nature of professions and professionalism has been the

---

**Box 1.3    Chief nursing officer's 10 key roles for nurses**

Order diagnostic investigations
Make and receive referrals direct
Admit and discharge patients for specified conditions and within agreed
    protocols
Manage patient caseloads
Run clinics e.g. ophthalmology or dermatology
Prescribe medications and treatments
Carry out a wide range of resuscitation procedures, including defibrillation
Perform minor surgery and outpatients procedures
Triage patients using the latest IT to the most appropriate health professional
Take a lead in the way local health services are organised and in the way
    they are run.

subject of much analysis, primarily in the sociological literature. In considering what a profession is Gomm (1996) reiterates the often quoted list of attributes or traits, which seemed to be a particular hallmark of sociologists studying the area prior to the 1970s (Roth 1974). The required traits tended to vary, but generally included a philosophy of public service and altruism, skills based on theoretical knowledge, extensive training or education, a code of conduct for practice and the issue of self-regulation. As Gomm (1996) and previous authors such as Jolley (1989) and Roth (1974) have noted, the degree to which such characteristics need to be present in order to be a profession is unclear and highly debatable. Roth's (1974) criticism of the trait approach is that it does not focus on the process of professionalisation, but on the product. This he argues, in itself is contaminated with the ideology and hopes of professional groups rather than an independent assessment of what they achieve (Roth 1974: 17). In reality, the concept may never be static, but reflects the changing needs of both society and those it serves. Freidson (1994) concluded that the term 'profession' lies in embracing it as an intrinsically ambiguous, multifaceted folk concept, of which no single definition or isolation of its essence will ever be generally persuasive.

To understand professions more fully, there is a need to consider the issues of power and context. This is because both of these factors can change over time, requiring the profession to adapt and become essentially metamorphic. Gomm (1996: 116) highlights the issue of power through the point that professionalism is about something 'that is claimed'. Such occupations monopolise an area of specialist knowledge. Within this monopolisation is a claim that their licence, usually a legislative right through act of parliament to do the specific work to the exclusion of others, and their mandate, the right to say how the work should be done, is in the public interest. There is a strong claim of altruism. Other writers, such as those from a Marxist perspective, examine professions through the degree to which they support the power structures of capitalist societies (Navarro 1976). The context is also important, because it is the society that enters into an agreement with the profession, an act of parliament being a clear example, who sanctions and allows the profession to function in its monopolistic way. However, as society changes and begins to view professions differently, there is a need for adaptation if the profession is both to maintain credibility and also keep many of the privileges of power it has accrued. The metamorphic nature of professions is one reason the trait approach appears too static as a definition.

In the issue of context, it's of value to briefly reconsider how the view of professions has altered in recent years. Prior to the 1970s, professions were seen in far more static concepts, defined by the aforementioned traits, espoused by authors such as Carr-Saunders and Wilson (1962). All other healthcare disciplines tended to revolve around and be judged against this concept, with nursing ultimately described as a 'semi-profession' (Etzioni 1969). Such value judgements presented the implicit message that medicine was the ideal and ultimate way to deliver healthcare, and all other disciplines were not quite as good. Such rigid boundaries remained uncriticised, with nursing periodically comparing itself to medicine in terms of its attempts to gain full professional status (Dalzell-Ward 1957; Powell 1963; Watkin 1956a, 1956b). In almost their entirety, such papers desired further trait related behaviour or evaluated how far the occupation had come in achieving their professionalising goal.

This predated the emergence of sociological writers such as Freidson (1970), Johnson (1972), Roth (1974) and Illich *et al.* (1977), who amongst others criticised the closed and, as they saw it, disabling effects in terms of power and control, of those they served. Roth (1974: 17) considered the 'attribute rating game' as an occupation's effort to increase its relative standing in the occupational world and to reap the attendant rewards. For Roth, sociologists who focus on attributes do not study the process, but participate in it. They have become the dupe of established professions and in his view, are arbitrators of occupations on the make. Roth's paper is a lively argument, reflective of several at the time, which argues that the traits of a profession so often cited, are largely a mixture of unproven, and indeed unexamined claims for professional control and autonomy. One of several examples he makes is the claim that a systematic body of theory requires a lengthy training. He questions whether it may in fact be the other way round. Quoting Freidson (1970), he argues that the content and length of training of an occupation, including abstract knowledge or theory, is frequently a product of a deliberate action of those who are trying to show that their occupation is a profession and should therefore be given autonomy (Freidson 1970: 79–80, cited by Roth 1974: 7).

However, professionalism can be used as a solution to various 'problems' involving occupations. Become a profession and the client need not worry about (an occupation's) competing interests because the client knows that the profession is obligated to be trustworthy. There will be a system of colleague control and a code of ethics to ensure members of the profession act ethically. This, as will be discussed, with reference to Sir Donald Irvine's speech was the trust that became damaged for the British public with the high profile cases involving the medical profession in the 1990s. In addition, if professions have an altruistic and service-orientated focus, with a professional code to supply their services to whoever needs it, then this can be countered by a body of evidence of the poor equity of service provision to women, the poor and ethnic minorities. The emergence of the National Service Frameworks (NSFs) in Britain in the late 1990s was one government initiated method to counter a lack of equity in health service provision. This criticism of the power professions wielded was summed up by Illich (1977: 17):

Merchants sell you the goods they stock. Guildsmen guarantee quality. Some craftspeople tailor their product to your measure or fancy. Professionals tell you what you need and claim the power to prescribe. They not only recommend what is good, but actually ordain what is right. Neither income, long training, delicate tasks nor social standing is the mark of the professional. Rather, it is his authority to define a person as client, to determine that person's need and to hand the person a prescription.

The extent to which the sociological theorists had an effect on altering professional structures and their relations with the public is questionable. The politics of the Thatcherite 1980s and their attack on the professions and the public sector was probably more significant. In many ways one might argue that right wing politics was borrowing the clothes of more left wing sociologists to add legitimacy to its arguments. What is clear however, is that for some time an alternative professional structure was not forthcoming. In utilising, Hugman (1991), Salvage (1985), Stacey (1992) and Williams (1993); Davies (1995) illustrates a more focussed critique of the professional pathway nursing was aiming to achieve in the 1980s. In addition, she offers a further analysis of the alternative approaches being discussed at the time. Jane Salvage (1985) had questioned nursing's desired traditional professional pathway and notably the wish for an all qualified nursing workforce. Such a desire ignored the reality of who was, and all through the history of modern nursing, who had been involved in performing basic nursing care. This was notably untrained people in and outside of the hospital. For Salvage this encapsulated the 'neglected' nursing auxiliary, although it is now recognised he/she has increasing access to a level of healthcare training. Salvage terms qualified nursing's, and notably in the mid-1980s the Royal College of Nursing's, lack of grasp on the reality of who performed much of the nursing care as 'the ostrich syndrome' (Salvage 1985: 86). In addition, such a uniform view imposed by this form of professionalism may not have reflected the reality that there were differing views and interests, and those, such as from students and managers could become submerged. Such an approach may meet the needs of the profession, but did it really address those of the healthcare system itself?

Davies (1995) explores what medical sociologist Margaret Stacey (1992: 257) terms 'new professionalism' based on the latter's work as a lay member of the General Medical Council (GMC). New professionalism focuses, notably in medicine, on the traditional concept of the one to one relationship with the patient. There needs to be both the recognition of the differing but equally valuable role of other healthcare professionals, and adjustments to the judgement and control over these other groups. This shift also includes an altered role in the power over the patient. The patient becomes, not necessarily first, 'but equal to and a part of the professional interest' (Stacey 1992: 260). Stacey argued that placing the patient above personal and sectional interests was certainly the ideal, but she felt under the old professionalism, it had not really worked out that way. Listening to and involving patients, and understanding how *they* see things, appear as the key to this changing professionalism.

It is important however, to fully acknowledge Davies' argument regarding gender and professionalism, because she raises issues which are relevant to the nurse-led clinic as it encroaches into the traditionally male-dominated area of medicine. Davies argues that in the criticism of professions the issue of gender has been largely ignored. In the development of professions, masculinity is an important issue, and historically medicine has been dominated by men and nursing by women. The irony or 'the twist' as Davies calls it, is that nursing is not a profession but an adjunct to a gendered concept of profession. This she suggests, means that nursing is the activity that enables medicine to present itself as masculine/rational, and to gain the power and privilege of doing so. Nursing's role may be not to become a profession in the present sense of the term, but to challenge the gendered basis of the concept. For medicine to function in this gendered, masculine vision, women's work has to be trivialised or devalued (Davies 1995). The issue here is how the nurse-led clinic retains many of the aspects of nursing – holistic care, the nurturing and caring aspects – yet challenges medicine by clearly acquiring many of the masculine, scientific aspects of that profession.

More recently, the former Chairman of the GMC, Sir Donald Irvine (2002), has quoted Margaret Stacey's work as an alternative professionalism for medicine. He identifies events in society such as the paediatric cardiac deaths at the Bristol Royal Infirmary and the serial killer and former GP Harold Shipman, as defining moments for medicine's relationship with the public, patients and the state. He believes patient experiences, expectations and choice have to be central to any new model of professionalism. In pragmatic terms, Irvine identifies the public stake in the GMC as having increased from 12 per cent to 25 per cent in 1994 and more recently to 40 per cent. He argues that team members in medicine need to learn and be open and honest about their professional performance, both together and individually. As part of their own internal clinical governance they should be using good data, collective audit and formative appraisal. Some doctors already think and practise this way, but others Irvine argues, see new quality measures as unnecessary bureaucratic impositions. They have not internalised them. He suggests that the better day to day internal governance is, through clinical teams or institutions such as the GMC, the lighter the external controls needed. It is the daily quality assurance of performance that matters to patients (Irvine 2002). Such a view from an elite member of the medical profession may well have been unheard of some 20 or so years ago, but it does demonstrate this necessary evolution of a profession. Also if the boundaries are moving, there is the potential for nursing to work with medicine in innovative ways, with respect for each other's skills, thus enhancing service provision.

Hugman (1991) and his examination of power in caring professions, is used by Davies (1995) to reinforce his concept of 'democratic professionalism'. Here the focus is in part on a greater equality in power and a reconsideration of the boundaries between the caring professions. Both the users and the professionals that often appear weak in the context of the hierarchies they encounter in healthcare, could in Hugman's ideal, foster partnerships and participation at the level of service delivery that are as visible as in anti-racist and anti-sexist struggles in health and welfare. Hugman argues that these areas show that the sharing of power is possible, where a common basis for understanding the experience of service users exists. Black-controlled services and services controlled by women can involve both professionals and service users, but they also offer concrete examples of how knowledge and skills can be shared (Hugman 1991). Such a view of democratic professionalism would require different relationships between professionals and service users, but also in the boundaries *between* the caring professions. This is naturally an area of significance in the emerging nurse-led clinics. However for Hugman, writing in 1991, he considered that without changes in existing forms of power, the prospect of greater unity amongst caring professions could have negative implications.

Williams (1993) in discussing changing professionalism, comes perhaps closest to what a nurse-led clinic can aim to achieve as part of its philosophy. This is particularly with a public suffering more chronic illness, and empowered through the media, the growth of support groups and the internet. For Williams, instead of the one way transmission of knowledge from the professional to the client, it becomes a two way transaction. This builds on the existing knowledge of the client, according to their needs and the professional's response to these. There is no longer a professional attempting to impose his or her view, the change is one 'from controlling to supporting and enabling' (Williams 1993: 12). This approach to education, based on the philosophy of the education of equals, poses a challenge to the way the professional's expert knowledge is viewed and utilised (Williams 1993). However, even with any changing boundaries, it is important not to believe that the issues of being professional, through respect, altruism and appropriate conduct cannot be disentangled from being a profession. They can and remain of paramount importance.

The critique of the concept of a profession that has occurred since the early 1970s allows preconceived ideas, often implicit and covert, to be exposed and challenged in the drive for better healthcare provision. Davies' (1995) central argument is that nursing is positioned as an adjunct to medicine, enabling it to function as it does. This issue of power and context can and should be applied to the emergence of the nurse-led clinic.

Why has medicine and indeed the Government, generally welcomed the nurse-led clinic? Is it because of the desperate need for a reduction in doctors' working hours? Is it to increase service access or is it the time-honoured fashion discussed by amongst others Hugman (1991) citing Howe (1986), of handing down the less specialist work to ancillary groups of sub professionals, 'ditching the dirty work', to enhance personal professionalism through higher status activities? The latter is an interesting argument, because it may be true of the medical consultant, focussing on highly specialised expertise, but in primary care, nurse-led clinics are encroaching on many areas of general medical practice, as well as challenging the gate-keeping role of the GP to health services and legitimised illness. Certainly when boundaries do appear to be changing between healthcare professions, the nursing press leap upon it as a cause for celebration (Oxtoby 2003). It's an area worth watching and importantly analysing, to make more explicit the issues surrounding nursing's own development.

These altering views of professionalism do tend to reinforce the aforementioned issue of empowerment within the nurse-led clinic, and a change of approach in caring for those living with illness and seeking the best possible quality of life. What will be of a continuing challenge is how to imbue this philosophy within the professional development of those who run nurse-led clinics. Time will tell whether history will repeat itself and hierarchical boundaries appear within the clinics, or they remain a partnership between provider and service user to augment the health experience. Current literature focuses on our approaches as healthcare professionals to involving the views of users to plan and assess the effectiveness of care (Anderson and Florin 2000; Anderson et al. 2002; Brooks and Gillam 2001; Gillespie et al. 2002).

Of interest has been the British Medical Association's (BMA) discussion paper regarding alternative methods of healthcare delivery between the professions (BMA 2002a). They termed this a 'ground breaking' new model for NHS care. Primarily, they emphasised the possibility of moving away from the general practitioner as the gatekeeper of access to healthcare, and utilising the nurse practitioner in primary care as the patient's first point of call, and the clinical nurse specialist in secondary care to coordinate services. The nurse practitioner could provide information and guide the patient to the relevant service. He/she would also deliver 'an expanded range of direct patient care' (BMA 2002a).

To some it may not be revolutionary, but it does discuss this powerful issue of the medical profession's dominance in gatekeeping to healthcare services. The impetus may be to free up medical time to deal with more serious conditions, rather than aiming to enhance the professional status of nursing. However, importantly, it is a document that attempts to provide the best service for the patient and their loved ones, through re-evaluating the healthcare team's skills. The press release for the document provided a new MORI poll of 1,972 adults aged 15 years and over at 198 sampling points in the UK (BMA 2002b). This noted that 87 per cent of people would be happy to see a nurse rather than a doctor, if their conditions were not serious. The document's omission to highlight the role of the nurse-led clinic in monitoring and maintaining optimum health in those with longstanding conditions, is offset by this encouraging figure.

## The changing philosophy of health education

The changing attitudes towards the traditional professional model coincided with altered views towards health education, which has always had a major role within nursing practice. Prior to the early 1980s the term 'health promotion' was unheard of, with 'health education' being the common term. This tended to represent all that encompassed the hierarchical approach to reducing potentially health damaging behaviour. Risk factors to health such as smoking, high cholesterol and obesity had been identified since the 1950s, and it seemed logical to inform or 'educate' patients to avoid these vices and live a healthier life.

But by 1980 the Black Report had been published in the UK linking poor health to lower social class (Townsend et al. 1992). This correlated sociological factors such as poor housing, low wages and income to the occurrence of a wide range of diseases and premature death. Such a reinforced view that medicine alone could not cure all ills, was augmented by the World Health Organization (WHO) in planning their health education programme for 1980–84. They realised that health education in isolation from other measures would not necessarily result in the radical changes required to herald a new era of improved health (Parish 1995). The prospect of health promotion as an alternative approach to improving a nation's health, became a key policy issue on the agenda of many nations in less than a decade, notably in the western, industrialised world (Parish 1995). Health promotion encompassed a wider view of improving health, which involved a variety of sociological factors and influences in planning health improvements. The importance of the patient or client as living and being a part of their environment, and not an uneducated vessel to be informed of their bad practices is an important philosophical change in health promotion. Such a change again links to this issue of enabling and supporting that should be a major part of the nurse-led clinic.

## The scope of professional practice

By 1992 the United Kingdom Central Council for Nursing and Midwifery (UKCC) had published the *Scope of Professional Practice* (UKCC 1992).

This document has been praised by many as a landmark publication, with Walsh (2001) arguing that the rapid development of the nurse practitioner in the UK occurred without the support of the UKCC, yet ironically without the *Scope of Professional Practice* it could never have occurred. The document was published at an appropriate time because in the years following, the concept of how we view and are seeing nursing services delivered has changed enormously.

The document placed the patient first by asking the practitioner not to be restricted by a traditional set of certificated 'extended' roles, but to reflect on developing their practice to offer the patient appropriate and holistic nursing care. It does seem to offer the nurse 'carte blanche' to do what they want provided they are deemed competent. But it is an adult document in loosening the traditional boundaries which may have restricted us from being innovative and offering more patient-focussed care. The previous relevant document had been the *Extended Role of the Nurse* circular from 1977 (DHSS 1977). This allowed extended roles if delegated by a doctor and deemed appropriate for nurses to carry out. But who judged the appropriateness? (Walsh 2001). By comparing the philosophies of these two documents, it is easy to see how the nurse-led clinics and services discussed in this chapter would have been hard pressed to have seen the light of day in previous years.

The 1977 document had seen the expansion of any nursing services as a mere set of skilled tasks, not as a holistic approach where the whole idea or philosophy of the service could be changed. In addition, the profession was portrayed as subservient to medicine. The *Scope of Professional Practice* as Walsh (2001) has explored, raised the issues of autonomy and accountability in developing skills. However, no nurse can be totally autonomous. This chapter itself has emphasised the nurse-led clinic as part of a team approach to care. It is the issues of independence and enjoying, as Walsh (2001) states, higher levels of autonomy that are the reality. It does also free nurses from the habit of collecting certificates for extended roles, which may not be accepted in other institutions. The skill(s) on the certificate may also not have been practised for some time, and this draws away from the concepts of reflection and continuing professional development, which are the cornerstone of competent practice.

## Advanced practice and who runs the nurse-led clinic?

In further exploring the concept of the nurse-led clinic it's worth considering how it links to advanced nurse practice, and how the practitioners running the clinics may be termed. Are they clinical nurse specialists, nurse consultants, practice nurses, nurse practitioners or advanced nurse practitioners?

The clinics themselves are simply what the title describes, they are nurse-led. Not all can be termed advanced practice, or run by the afore-mentioned groups. An example could be the pre-operative clinic. Patients may be seen in a clinic, perhaps a week before admission for surgery, and the nurse explains the operative procedure and associated care. He/she offers to show the patient the ward or unit, including the intensive care unit, and allay fears of the unknown for patient and loved ones. At this point routine and any specialist bloods, together with a chest X-ray may be taken. Health promotion advice can be offered, including how the person should care for themselves on returning home, and questions and concerns answered. The nurse is then in the position to discuss with colleagues any encountered problems, such as poor skin condition or diagnosed respiratory problems that may affect the more usual plan of care or skill mix of staff.

Such a clinic is a vital and much needed part of the care of the patient, but may not be termed advanced practice. However, with the advent and rapid growth of many of the clinics described in this chapter, advanced nurse practice is clearly a significant part of the nurse-led clinic and the practitioners involved. Advanced practice as a term is in itself somewhat nebulous. Its definition does appear to alter depending on whom you ask, together with views on the appropriate level of educational preparation. The RCN advises that specific nurse practitioner education should be at a minimum of first degree level. All RCN accredited higher education institutions for nurse practitioner preparation offer Bachelor level preparation, and in some cases Masters level too. Indeed, increasingly in the UK, education for this role is also being offered at Masters level through Higher Education Institutions.

Cox (2001) provided a useful definition when comparing the work of an advanced nurse practitioner to that of the United States physician's assistant. The former possesses advanced assessment, diagnostic, prescriptive and technological skills with an acute care and primary care focus. 'The advanced nurse practitioner provides comprehensive health/illness management, consultancy and primary care in a variety of clinical settings ... (they) can work independently, managing a caseload of patients without supervision, or in a team that is consultant led' (Cox 2001: 169).

The clinical nurse specialist (CNS) remains more actively involved in caring for hospitalised patients, although as Cox and Ahluwalia (2001) identify, they can be found in the patient clinic environment. The multi-faceted roles that may be commonly associated with the CNS include educator, researcher, consultant, expert practitioner and change agent. The nurse consultant is clearly seen in running nurse-led clinics, as the closing chapters in this text testify. However, their role also encompasses the generation of research and implementing this as part of their role in leading, advancing and changing practice. Practice nurses outside of the hospital environment are again part of the nursing team involved in running nurse-led clinics. In the primary care environment, their employment has more than doubled in England from 4,632 to 10,689 between 1989 and 1999 (DOH 2000c). By 2001 there were considered to be 18,500 practice nurses in the UK, the largest 'branch' of community nursing (BMA 2001). Reducing the working hours of GPs, who may not be able to see patients for several days, is an impetus for the expansion of nursing roles, but as Baraniak (2001) states above, this impetus can come from a re-evaluation of who it is most appropriate for the patient to see. This is as opposed to long entrenched traditional practice boundaries.

The role most closely associated to the advancing practice of the nurse-led clinic, is that of the nurse practitioner, sometimes termed the advanced nurse practitioner. The addition of this word, both separates their role from all registered nurses who may be termed a 'nurse practitioner' and also indicates the advancement of their practice to a higher level. The irony of this of course, is that until recently there has been no credible move towards regulation of the specialist or advanced practice role and hence that of the nurse practitioner. Changes have now occurred with the NMC alterations to the nursing and midwifery register (NMC 2003). Therefore previously there was in fact no marker to be able to make clear judgements regarding the classification of nursing roles. The association of nurse-led clinics to the nurse practitioner's role may come from the fact that both areas have developed side by side in the UK through the 1980s and beyond.

The definition of the nurse practitioner in the UK has been influenced strongly by the development of the role in the United States. The term first appeared in 1965 at the University of Colorado. A project developed by Dr Henry Silver, a physician and Dr Loretta Ford, a nurse, was concerned with the increasing population of the US, but a limited number of primary care physicians (Stilwell 1988). Subsequently, the two developed a four-month programme for nurses, which included the skills of physical assessment. The course focussed on childcare, and offered nurses the skills to appraise acute and chronic conditions, including appropriate referral, evaluation and the temporary management of emergency situations until medical assistance was available (Silver *et al.* 1967). In addition, was the development of a Master's degree programme for nurse practitioner training by Physician Eugene Stead and Thelma Inglis, a nurse. This met with some resistance, and was not accredited by The National League of Nursing until 1977. This was due to the extension into what were felt to be inappropriate medical tasks that may be unsafe (Fisher and Horowitz 1977). The role of the physician's assistant also developed in the mid-1960s, linked in part to the practise of Vietnam war veterans, with the first training programme at Duke University in North

Carolina. Both nurse practitioners and physician's assistants co-exist today.

The development of the nurse practitioner role in the US could be seen as a response to society's changing health needs, and medicine's inability to deal with simple medical problems (Stilwell 1988). This was believed to stem from the shortage of physicians in general medical practice. Ford and Silver have provided other reasons for developing the role, including the former's desire to test an expanded scope of practice for nurses, and the latter's interest in improving child healthcare (Pearson 1985). In addition, the government's interest in funding these courses was also likely to have reflected a need to contain rising healthcare costs (Stilwell 1988). The term and concept of the nurse practitioner arrived in the UK in the early 1980s. Much of this was through the work of Barbara Stilwell (Bowling and Stilwell 1988; Stilwell 1984, 1985a, 1985b). The RCN Institute commenced the first programme in the UK for nurse practitioners in 1990, moving from diploma to a degree level course in 1996.

In their definitions of the nurse practitioner both Stilwell (1988) and Walsh (2001) draw on the work of Bliss and Cohen (1977). This definition includes the ability to assess the health status of individuals and their families, through health and medical history taking, physical examination and the defining of health and developmental problems. In addition, are the skills of instituting and providing continuity of healthcare to clients, working with the client to ensure understanding of and compliance with the therapeutic regime within established protocols, and recognition of when to refer the client to a physician or other healthcare provider.

The definition also emphasises the areas highlighted above in the role of the nurse-led clinic, namely providing health promotion and the philosophical shift to increasingly involving clients in planning for their healthcare. The increased autonomy for the nurse is leavened by a need to work in collaboration with other healthcare providers to provide and coordinate services (Bliss and Cohen 1977). The term 'advanced practice nurse' is defined by the American Nursing Association (ANA 1996) to cover four roles of which the nurse practitioner is one. The others include the CNS, nurse–midwife and nurse–anaesthetist. Advanced practice nurse's skills include: managing patients to a greater depth and breadth of knowledge, skills and competencies; practising with greater autonomy; exercising a high degree of independent judgement and well developed communication skills with multidisciplinary teams across complex healthcare environments (ANA 1996).

The RCN Council defined the nurse practitioner and an appropriate educational preparation in 1995, this was updated to reflect the evolution of the role in 2002 (RCN 2002). This definition is similar to those described, with an emphasis on the autonomy of the role, in addition to counselling and health education skills. Importantly, the definition emphasises the supportive role in helping people to manage and live with illness, and the receiving of patients with undifferentiated and undiagnosed problems (RCN 2002).

The difficulty in the confusing array of terms for nurses in practice is recognised within the profession (Gulland 2002). For the vulnerable public it can be a minefield. London South Bank University has produced literature for primary care teams who need to decide which of their programmes would be most appropriate to the patients' and practice needs (SBU 2002). This may be a community health care specialist practitioner (general practice nurse), including modules in minor illness, or nurse practitioner preparation. The literature in fact recognises the overlap in places, such as the management of minor illness, chronic disease management and the assessment of health needs. The practice nurse route primarily focuses on developing the knowledge and skills commensurate with taking responsibility for the total practice nursing services provided by the practice. The nurse practitioner course primarily focuses on clinical skills development to enable nurses to make a diagnosis and implement appropriate care as part of their autonomous role, for a wide range of patient presentations across the age range (SBU 2002). The issues surrounding advanced nursing practice can be further explored in Woods (2000).

## The evidence for the effectiveness of nurse-led clinics

There is increasing evidence that expanding nurse-led services are comparable and in some cases better in terms of patient satisfaction, quality and cost, to those that are medically led. It's important to note that comparison of nurse practitioners to doctors, cannot necessarily be used as an indicator of the effectiveness of nurse-led clinics. This is because the role of the nurse practitioner is not defined solely by the running of clinics; the accident and emergency nurse practitioner being a clear example. However, nurse practitioner services have been generally well evaluated in research studies (Horrocks et al. 2002; Kinnersley et al. 2000; Mundinger et al. 2000). In addition, Shum et al. (2000) positively evaluated nurse-led management of minor illnesses in general practice by practice nurses.

Those studies examining nurse-led clinics have usually focussed on highly specific services (Hill 1997; Ridsdale et al. 1997; Sharples et al. 2002). For Ridsdale et al. (1997) a randomised controlled trial involving a nurse-led clinic for the management of epilepsy in general practice noted that the service could significantly improve the level of advice and drug management recorded. Sharples et al. (2002) noted little difference between the services provided by doctors and nurses in clinics for managing chronic respiratory disease. However, it was highlighted that the nurse-led clinics were more costly, with higher numbers of patients admitted by the nurse to hospital, longer consultations and significantly more antibiotics prescribed. Subsequently, it was seen that in the two years of the study, doctor-led care remained at a steady cost, while nurse-led care reduced. This was suggestive of a learning curve for the nurses, and a predicted reduced cost in the future of the service.

The setting up of any nurse-led clinic, needs to incorporate a system for measuring worth. This is particularly important while this new way of service delivery establishes itself, and while the skills of nurses is so variable. Measurement will occur through varying forms. Patient satisfaction alone may be only a part of the whole picture. If nurse-led clinics can offer easier access to a healthcare practitioner and longer consultation times, a cynic could argue that satisfaction would rise. Chapter 4 explores the variety of research methods available to capture the worth of the clinic being provided. Chapter 2 considers the vital issues of professional development and measuring competence. These are necessary to not only provide a quality service, but to protect the public and the nurses themselves. Competence and confidence do not necessarily go hand in hand.

At this early stage it is worth considering the differences between the terms 'clinical audit' and 'evaluation'. Essentially there is some overlap in the terms, and indeed interpretation can differ. Clinical audit is currently fashionable as a method of improving and maintaining quality care and is seen as an ongoing process of development (Morrell and Harvey 1999). It can be defined as a quality improvement process that seeks to improve patient care and outcomes through a systematic review of care against explicit criteria, together with the implementation of change (NICE 2002).

The clinical audit cycle contains a variety of elements which will include questioning what is it we are trying to achieve, sampling, questioning whether it is being achieved through a variety of data collection methods and benchmarking. The latter is the comparison of performance criteria against what is considered best practice. It is often termed as comparison against the best equivalent provider (Morrell and Harvey 1999). The benchmarks created for practice comparison need to be realistic and these can often be generated nationally. The cycle is completed by making appropriate changes and then questioning whether this has made things better (NICE 2002).

Evaluation is slightly different, although it can be a part of clinical audit. What is important is to consider both elements. Evaluation assesses 'merit' or 'worth'. It is asking those who run nurse-led clinics, to consider beyond the quality, the actual value of the service they provide. Merely seeing an increased number of patients, or providing high standard advice, support or manipulation of medication is an admirable service, but evaluation provides consideration of the outcomes, which indicate whether this is of any value. Chapter 4 offers further guidance in the issue of measuring effectiveness, and the differing value judgements that can emerge from utilising areas such as patient perceptions, and the quantitative and qualitative research paradigms.

In conclusion, this chapter has explored the emergence of the nurse-led clinic and the suggested reasons as to why their proliferation has occurred at this time point. The Labour Government's support of nurse-led services generally, has encouraged innovation across the wide spectra of this practice area. This has notably been through the PMS sites and NHS walk-in centres. Such support continues to indicate a need to ensure that nurse-led clinics provide a measurably high quality service, through the appropriate use of research application. The former lack of a move to regulate roles within the domain of specialist and advanced practice nursing, raises concern that those running nurse-led clinics should be able to demonstrate competence, and that this is part of ongoing professional development. Adequate support from the nursing profession itself to safeguard the practice of those who push the boundaries of healthcare delivery is a mandatory requirement.

## References

Alderman, C. (1997) 'Anticipating anxiety' (a nurse-led pre-admission clinic within a gynaecology unit), *Nursing Standard* 12(1), 22–23.

American Nursing Association (1996) *Scope and Standards of Advanced Practice Registered Nursing*, American Nursing Association.

Anderson, W. and Florin, D. (2000) *Involving the Public – One of Many Priorities*, London: The King's Fund.

Anderson, W., Florin, D., Gillam, S. and Mountford, L. (2002) *Every Voice Counts*, London: The King's Fund.

Baraniak, C. (2001) 'A normal community', *Primary Health Care* 11(2), 14.

Baraniak, C. and Gardner, L. (2001) 'Nurse-led General Practice – the implications of nurse-led practice for nurses, doctors and patients', in Lewis, R., Gillam, S. and Jenkins, C. (eds) *Personal Medical Services Pilots: Modernising Primary Care?* London: The King's Fund, pp. 75–87.

Binnie, A., Perkins, J. and Hands, L. (1999) 'Exercise and nursing therapy for patients with intermittent claudication', *Journal of Clinical Nursing* 8(2), 190–200.

Blair, T., Prime Minister (2000) 'Tony Blair's speech to the House of Commons on NHS Modernisation', 22 March 3.30 pm.

Bliss, A.A. and Cohen, E.D. (eds) (1977) *The New Health Professionals*, Maryland: Aspen Systems Corporation.

Bowling, A. and Stilwell, B. (eds) (1988) *The Nurse: Practice Nurses and Nurse Practitioners in Primary Health Care in Family Practice*, London: Scutari Press.

British Medical Association (2001) *Practice Nursing (September 2001)*, a discussion paper by the GPC's Practice Nurse Working Group, London: BMA.

British Medical Association (2002a) *A Future Model for the Healthcare Workforce*, Discussion Paper 9, London: BMA.

British Medical Association (2002b) 'A New Model for NHS Care. 28 February', press release, London: BMA.

Brooks, F. and Gillam, S. (2001) *New Beginnings*, London: The King's Fund.

Carr-Saunders, A.M. and Wilson, P.A. (1962) *The Professions*, London: Oxford University Press.

Cox, C.L. (2001) 'Advanced Nurse Practitioners and Physician Assistants: What is the difference? Comparing the USA and UK', *Hospital Medicine* 62(3), 169–171.

Cox, C.L. and Ahluwalia, S. (2001) 'Clinical effectiveness, nursing diagnosis and the role of the clinical nurse specialist and nurse practitioner', in Cox, C.L. and Reyes-Hughes, A. (eds) *Clinical Effectiveness in Practice*, Houndmills, Basingstoke: Palgrave.

Dalzell-Ward, A.J. (1957) 'The reason and need for professional organisations', *Nursing Mirror* 8 November, 431–432.

Davies, C. (1995) *Gender and the Professional Predicament in Nursing*, Buckingham: Open University Press.

Denning, J. (2000) 'A nurse-led clinic for peritoneal dialysis', *Nursing Times* 96(13), 44–45.

Department of Health and Social Security (1977) *The Extended Role of the Nurse*, London: DHSS.

Department of Health (1989) *Report of the Advisory Group on Nurse Prescribing (The Crown Report)*, London: DOH.

Department of Health (1997) *The NHS (Primary Care) Act*, London: DOH.

Department of Health (1998) *The Crown Report. A Report on the Supply and Administration of Medicines Under Group Protocols*, London: DOH.

Department of Health (1999a) *Review of Prescribing, Supply and Administration of Medicines. Final Report (Crown II Report)*, London: DOH.

Department of Health (1999b) *Making a Difference: Strengthening the Nursing, Midwifery and Health Visiting Contribution to Health and Healthcare*, London: DOH.

Department of Health (2000a) *Health Service Circular 2000/026. Patient Group Directions (England only)*, London: DOH.

Department of Health (2000b) *The National Service Framework for Coronary Heart Disease*, London: DOH.

Department of Health (2000c) *Statistical Bulletin – Statistics for General Medical Practitioners in England 1989–1999*, London: DOH.

Department of Health (2002) *Primary Care Act, Personal Medical Services (PMS) Pilots. National Evaluation of First Wave NHS Personal Medical Service Pilots*, London: DOH.

Etzioni, A. (1969) *The Semi-Professions and Their Organisation*, New York: Free Press.

Fisher, D.W. and Horowitz, S.M. (1977) 'The Physician's Assistant: profile of a new health professional', in Bliss, A.A. and Cohen, E.D. (eds) *The New Health Professionals*, Maryland: Aspen Systems Corporation.

Freidson, E. (1970) *Profession of Medicine: A Study of the Sociology of Applied Knowledge*, Chicago: University of Chicago Press.

Freidson, E. (1994) *Professionalism Reborn: Theory, Prophecy and Policy*, Cambridge: Polity Press.

Gardner, L. (1998) 'Does nurse-led care mean second-class care?' *Nursing Times* 9(94), 50–51.

Gillespie, R., Florin, D. and Gillam, S. (2002) *Changing Relationships: Findings of the Patient Involvement Project*, London: The King's Fund.

Gomm, R. (1996) 'Professions and professionalism', in Aitken, V. and Jellicoe, H. (eds) *Behavioural Sciences for Health Professionals*, London: Saunders, pp. 115–121.

Gulland, A. (2002) 'Making advances', *Nursing Times* 98(33), 10.

Hatchett, R. (2000) 'The emergence of the nurse-led clinic: a qualitative study with recommendations for practice development', unpublished MSc dissertation, London: City University.

Hill, J. (1997) 'Patient satisfaction in a nurse-led rheumatology clinic', *Journal of Advanced Nursing* 25, 347–354.

Horrocks, S., Anderson, E. and Salisbury, C. (2002) 'Systematic review of whether Nurse Practitioners working in primary care can provide equivalent care to doctors', *British Medical Journal* 324, 819–823.

Howe, D. (1986) *Social Workers and Their Practice in Welfare Bureaucracies*, Aldershot: Gower Publishing Ltd.

Hugman, R. (1991) *Power in the Caring Professions*, London: Macmillan.

Illich, I., Zola, I.K., McKnight, J., Caplan, J. and Shaiken, H. (1977) *Disabling Professions*, New York: Marion Boyars.

Illich, I. (1977) 'Disabling professions', in Illich, I., Zola, I.K., McKnight, J., Caplan, J. and Shaiken, H. (eds) *Disabling Professions*, New York: Marion Boyars, pp. 11–39.

Irvine, D. (2002) *Patients, Doctors and the Public Interest. DARE Lecture 2002*, given as part of the Faculty of Public Health Medicine Annual Scientific Meeting, Southport.

Johnson, T.J. (1972) *Professions and Power*, London: Macmillan Press Ltd.

Jolley, M. (1989) 'The professionalisation of nursing: an uncertain path', in Jolley, M. and Allan, P. (eds) *Current Issues in Nursing*, London: Chapman & Hall, pp. 1–22.

Kinnersley, P., Anderson, E., Parry, K., Clement, J., Archard, L. and Turton, P. (2000) 'Randomised controlled trial of nurse practitioner versus general practitioner care for patients requesting "same day" consultations in primary care', *British Medical Journal* 320, 1043–1048.

Lewis, R. (2001) *Nurse led Primary Care: Learning from PMS Pilots*, London: The King's Fund.

Maclaine, K. (1998) 'Clarifying higher level roles in nursing practice', *Professional Nurse* 14(3), 159–163.

Milburn, A, Rt. Hon, Secretary of State for Health (2000) Speech to Royal College of Nursing Annual Congress, 5 April, transcript held in London: The Royal College of Nursing Library.

Moore, A. (1999) 'Bumpy Ride, But on Course', *Nursing Standard* 13(27), 18–19.

Morrell, C. and Harvey, G. (1999) *The Clinical Audit Handbook: Improving the Quality of Health Care*, London: Bailliere Tindall and the Royal College of Nursing.

Muir, J. and Burnett, C. (1999) 'Setting up a nurse-led clinic for intractable childhood constipation', *British Journal of Community Nursing* 4(8), 395–399.

Mundinger, M.O., Kane, R.L., Lenz, E.R. *et al.* (2000) 'Primary care outcomes in patients treated by Nurse Practitioners or Physicians: a randomized trial', *Journal of the American Medical Association* 283(1), 59–68.

National Institute for Clinical Excellence (2002) *Principles for Best Practice in Clinical Audit*, Abingdon, Oxon: Radcliffe Medical Press.

Navarro, V. (1976) *Medicine Under Capitalism*, London: Croom Helm.

Newton, V. (1996) 'Care in pre-admission clinics', *Nursing Times* 92(1), 27–28.

Nursing and Midwifery Council (2003) 'NMC confirms details of new three-part register', NMC press statement 7 March. www.nmc-uk.org.

Office for National Statistics (2002) 'The Big Number', 30 September. www. statistics.gov.uk/releases.

Oxtoby, K. (2003) 'Let's work together', *Nursing Times* 99(4), 23–26.

Parish, R. (1995) 'Health promotion: rhetoric and reality', in Bunton, R., Nettleton, S. and Burrows, R. (eds) *The Sociology of Health Promotion*, London: Routledge, pp. 13–23.

Pearson, L. (1985) 'Perspectives 20 years later from the pioneers of the NP movement', *Nurse Practitioner* 10, 10–15.

Powell, M.B. (1963) 'The fundamental problem in nursing', *Nursing Times* 11 October, 1299–1300.

Ridsdale, L., Robins, D., Cryer, C. and Williams, H. (1997) 'Feasibility and effects of nurse run clinics for patients with epilepsy in general practice: randomised controlled trial', *British Medical Journal* 314, 120–122.

Roe, B., Walsh, N. and Huntington, J. (2001) *Breaking the Mould: Nurses Working in PMS Pilots*, Project Report No. 19, Birmingham: Health Service Management Centre.

Roth, J.A. (1974) 'Professionalism: the sociologist's decoy', *Sociology of Work and Occupations* 1(1), 6–23.

Royal College of Nursing (2002) *Competencies in Nursing: Nurse Practitioners – an RCN Guide to the Nurse Practitioner Role, Competencies and Programme Accreditation*, London: RCN, July.

Ryan, C. (2000) 'GPs slam "favours" for nurse-led centre', *Nursing Times* 96(45), p. 6.

Ryan, P. (2000) 'The benefits of a nurse-led pre-operative assessment clinic', *Nursing Times* 96(39), 42–43.

Salvage, J. (1985) *The Politics of Nursing*, London: Heinemann.

SBU (2002) BSc (Hons)/PG Dip Community Health Care Specialist Practitioner (General Practice Nursing) or RCN Accredited BSc (Hons) Nurse Practitioner (Primary Health Care)? London: South Bank University.

Sharples, L.D., Edmunds, J., Bilton, D. *et al.* (2002) 'A randomized controlled crossover trial of nurse practitioner versus doctor led outpatient care in a bronchiectasis clinic', *Thorax* 57(8), 661–666.

Shum, C., Humphreys, A., Wheeler, D. *et al.* (2000) 'Nurse management of patients with minor illnesses in General Practice: MultiCentre Randomised Controlled Trial', *British Medical Journal* 320, 1038–1043.

Silver, H.K., Ford, L.C. and Stearly, S.G. (1967) 'A program to increase health care for children – the Paediatric Nurse Practitioner Program', *Paediatrics* 39, 756–760.

Stacey, M. (1992) *Regulating British Medicine: The General Medical Council*, Chichester: Wiley.

Stilwell, B. (1984) 'The nurse in practice', *Nursing Mirror* 158(21), 17–22.

Stilwell, B. (1985a) 'The Nurse Practitioner – 1. Setting the scene', *Nursing Mirror* 160(15), 15–16.

Stilwell, B. (1985b) 'The Nurse Practitioner – 2. An unlikely setting (Nurse Practitioners in the Bronx)', *Nursing Mirror* 160(16), 15–16.

Stilwell, B. (1988) 'The origins and development of the Nurse Practitioner role – a worldwide perspective', in Bowling, A. and Stilwell, B. (eds) *The Nurse: Practice Nurses and Nurse Practitioners in Primary Health Care, in Family Practice*, London: Scutari Press, pp. 3–12.

Townsend, P., Davidson, N. and Whitehead, M. (1992) *Inequalities in Health: The Black Report and The Health Divide*, Harmondsworth: Penguin Books.

UKCC (1992) *The Scope of Professional Practice*, London: United Kingdom Central Council (available through the Nursing and Midwifery Council, London).

Vowden, K. (1997) 'Leg ulcer management in a nurse-led, hospital based clinic', *Journal of Wound Care* 6(5), 233–236.

Wallis, L. (2000) 'Back to basics' (a nurse-led clinic for people with back pain at North Tees General Hospital), *Nursing Standard* 14(17), 14–15.

Walsh, M. (2000) *Nursing Frontiers: Accountability and the Boundaries of Care*, Oxford: Butterworth-Heinemann.

Walsh, M. (2001) 'The Nurse Practitioner and hospital-based care: setting the scene', in *Nurse Practitioners: Developing the Role in Hospital Settings*, Oxford: Butterworth-Heinemann, pp. 3–11.

Watkin, V. (1956a) 'The professional status of hospital nurses – 1', *Nursing Times* 15 June, 545–546.

Watkin, V. (1956b) 'The professional status of hospital nurses – 2', *Nursing Times* 29 June, 600–601.

Williams, J. (1993) 'What is a profession? Experience versus expertise', in Walmsley, J., Reynolds, J., Shakespeare, P. and Woolfe, R. (eds) *Health, Welfare and Practice: Reflecting on Roles and Relationships*, London: Sage.

Woods, L.P. (2000) *The Enigma of Advanced Nursing Practice*, Salisbury, Wilts: Quay Books.

## Chapter 2

# Professional development in the nurse-led clinic

*Richard Hatchett*

This chapter explores perhaps one of the most important areas of the nurse-led clinic, the issue of professional development. The term is used here in preference to that of education or training. Professional development certainly encompasses education, but the former term emphasises the underlying philosophy that learning needs to be ongoing and developmental. No nurse will work in a clinic having acquired all of the necessary skills before practising. Many skills will be brought to the post, but will also need to be added to, developed further, updated and in many cases reassessed for competency to ensure that they remain at an appropriately high standard. Training has always been a term I personally dislike, because it does represent moulding someone through repetition, rather than developing practice appropriate to differing patient needs. It does however, seem to belong more to an era where education was seen as the passage of knowledge from someone who knew, to someone who didn't, and who required moulding to a rather narrow and focussed way of doing things. It also appears rather synonymous with the traditional approach to professional education, as discussed in the opening chapter, with a single period of intense learning, and the protection of specialist knowledge. This chapter will emphasise the need to actively share knowledge among colleagues as healthcare providers, and indeed the need to learn from the client or patient themselves.

Throughout the chapter various methods of learning are explored, including clinical supervision and reflection. The suggestion is made of the need to move away from pure classroom teaching and 'going away' on courses. This is because courses may achieve increased participants' awareness and motivation to change the way they work through increased knowledge, but may do little to help practitioners deal with the barriers they face on returning to work when they try and implement their new-found knowledge. This can therefore be regarded as the focus of clinical supervision and action learning. Courses such as those that incorporate physical assessment, pharmacology and legal aspects *are* strongly emphasised here, but in conjunction with the continued recognition of an ongoing approach to learning in the clinical area. The reality is also that staff are finding it increasingly difficult to be released from the work environment, and techniques such as work based and distance learning are emerging, together with clinical supervision as viable methods to enhance professional development. As will be highlighted, measuring the actual effectiveness of techniques such as clinical supervision and reflection in augmenting practice through assessment has produced some debate, although little formal research has been undertaken on linking these processes to outcomes in practice. Throughout the chapter quotes will be included from a series of interviews undertaken for this book, with practitioners who run nurse-led clinics and managers involved in the overall service.

The main aim of professional development in the nurse-led clinic, and indeed in all areas of nursing, is to protect the public against dangerous practice and to avoid the delivery of a sub-standard service. Professional development differs from practice development in that the focus is on the nurse rather than the patient, although both are interrelated (Manley 2001). At the present time any nurse can run a nurse-led clinic, and the role of the nurse practitioner, many of whom undertake such clinics, was only during 2003 beginning to move towards specific regulation via the Nursing and Midwifery Council (NMC) (NMC 2003). This meant that any registered nurse had been able to call themselves a nurse practitioner, running nurse-led clinics and practising what may be termed advanced practice skills. However, it should be emphasised that the NMC had previously set out to protect the public by the development of higher level of practice standards, and regarded these standards as the gateway to becoming a consultant nurse.

The document the *Scope of Professional Practice* originally published in 1992, offers an element of public protection. This places the patient first by asking the practitioner not to be restricted by a traditional set of certificated 'extended' roles, but to reflect on developing their practice to offer the patient the best possible appropriate and holistic nursing care within an ongoing competency framework. This emphasis incorporates the need to ensure that whoever is carrying out the skills of care is competent to do so (UKCC 1992). However, the emphasis is on self-assessment and self-regulation. There can therefore be the potential for, or actual problem of, what may be termed 'unconscious incompetence', that is being unaware that elements of your practice are not competent. The question also arises whether confidence and competence always go hand in hand, and whether the nurse can sometimes undertake a task or skill to save time, or through hierarchical pressure, that they may not be fully competent to do. Reflective practice may be useful here, as it can enable practitioners to develop their self-knowledge so that action follows from this, rather than coercion or the demands of others.

A 1994 survey commissioned by the Department of Health examined the interface between junior hospital doctors and ward nurses (Greenhalgh & Co 1994). The aim was to improve patient care by exploring what activities junior doctors and nurses undertook, with the ultimate view of ascertaining which skills could be suitably transferred to nurses. The detailed research included visits to ten clinical areas and 266 postal questionnaires. It appeared that 87.5 per cent of 24 wards chosen as case studies, offered nurses appropriate personal education and/or certification when they undertook additional skills. From the questionnaires 81 per cent of employing authorities appeared to do the same. The additional duties included taking a patient history, venous blood sampling, insertion of a peripheral intravenous cannula, referring a patient for an investigation, and writing discharge letters to general practitioners (GPs) and other doctors.

However, education appeared to fall into the traditional approach of one-off learning and testing, with the latter not occurring on a periodic basis. Some wards reported that no routine testing of the skill took place at all, where on others it took place annually as part of the individual performance review (IPR). Occasionally this was on an even more regular basis by the ward sister/charge nurse or nurse manager. Only 50 per cent of the 24 wards reported that competency testing was always or usually undertaken. It would also be interesting to note how this differed from medical colleagues' preparation. Nurses were trusted to adhere to the *Scope of Professional Practice* and only undertake activities for which they had been suitably prepared or in which they felt competent (Greenhalgh & Co 1994: 78).

Yet as described throughout this book, nurse-led clinics frequently involve the use and development of clinical skills not traditionally in the domain of nursing practice. Many of these fall into the area of advanced practice. It is important here not to equate advanced nursing practice with undertaking medical interventions. Manley (1996) reinforces the view that advanced practice is about advancing the practice of nursing, not medicine, within the context of organisations. There is the need to avoid the danger that the core nursing attributes are replaced by core medical ones. The definition of advanced practice has been discussed in Chapter One, and differs depending on which organisation's criteria you refer to. It can be a confusing area with Cox (2001) providing one definition when comparing the work of an advanced nurse practitioner to that of the United States Physician's Assistant. The former is defined by Cox (2001) as being educated to Masters level and possessing advanced assessment, diagnostic, prescriptive and technological skills with an acute care and primary care focus: 'The advanced nurse practitioner provides comprehensive health/illness management, consultancy and primary care in a variety of clinical settings ... (they) can work independently, managing a caseload of patients without supervision, or in a team that is consultant. This presumably could be medical or nurse consultant led' (Cox 2001: 169).

The physician's assistant has received a broad education in medicine at Masters degree level, and is licensed in a state or credentialised by a federal employer to practise medicine under the direct supervision of a doctor. They will provide a broad range of medical and surgical care in a variety of clinical settings that is traditionally performed by a doctor. They work as a member of a team with their supervising doctor as the leader of the team (Cox 2001). Their role includes undertaking physical examinations, diagnosing and treating illnesses, ordering and interpreting tests, through to counselling on preventative healthcare, assisting in surgery and in many states prescribing medications (Cox 2001). The aspect of maintaining nursing attributes may be an issue to some, but the Physician's Assistant is not always a nurse. In discussion with both Professor Carol Cox and Barbara Stilwell, the latter as one of the pioneers of nurse practitioners in the UK, advanced practice is as much the development of cognitive ability as practical skills. These extracts are taken directly from the interview transcripts:

> I think that in the main, the real element in relation to advanced practice, is that this is a practitioner who is working independently, and that you mentioned a minute ago about a caseload, but it's how the practitioner manages that caseload, the clinical decision making, the critical decision making associated with the management of the patient within that particular caseload.... What you see in advanced practice is a very highly proficient, accomplished clinician, who is able to critically analyse what is going on with the patient and prescribe appropriate care that is culturally specific, if I can use that, for that particular patient. In other words they are sensitive to the needs of the patient.
>
> (Cox 2002)

> I have a, I have to confess upfront really, that I have quite an existential view of advanced nurse practice, rather than a practical one, and that's because I think that when a nurse has a consultation, like anybody else, like any other person who has a consultation, the consultation kind of, is a lived experience between those people ... it's happening right there, in the present moment, and what the nurse has to use her/his skills to do, I think, is to find out what's actually going on in that consultation, to find out what the meaning of that consultation is for that patient, as well as what's the meaning for the nurse, for herself/himself. And because she/he has the skills to discover that information, what she/he can do is to prioritise, what has to be dealt with as she/he sees it, and to check that out with the patient. So, you

know, what she/he's looking at, is to say what's going to be the most urgent thing I have to do in this consultation, and then checking out what she sees as her reality, is actually what the patient also sees as the reality, and to explore those avenues.

(Stilwell 2002)

These extracts emphasise the need for a critical thinking and skills based learning approach, beyond that which the more usual education for nurse registration offers at the present time. Both also demonstrate highly developed nursing skills, such as sensitivity to the patient, understanding the world through the patient's eyes and patient preferences. In addition, changes in practice can occur rapidly and sometimes in an unpredictable way, with the increasing need to meet quality standards and create a workload that's more equitable amongst healthcare professionals. Therefore, in developing practice there is a need to be politically sensitive, and anticipate changes on the horizon which will alter service provision and education needs.

## Education and protecting the public

In considering the protection of the public, it remains highly unlikely that the concept of the nurse-led clinic will become subject to specific educational requirements or a set of practice competencies. The simple reason being that it is a broad service rather than a more specific role. There have been more recent debates regarding the regulation of the role of the nurse practitioner, many of whom run nurse-led clinics. This is primarily because of the specific utilisation of advanced practice skills in areas such as patient history taking, managing those with differential, often undiagnosed conditions, and in critical thinking skills. The latter may be used in areas such as deciding whether the nurse practitioner has the skills to address the patient's problems, choosing an appropriate treatment or medication in partnership with the patient, or appropriately referring to another healthcare professional.

For the nurse practitioner the simple answer would seem to be protection of the role and title under NMC regulation, which there is now a move towards (NMC 2003). This would ideally stipulate that to practise as a nurse practitioner a specific educational pathway, but more pragmatically particularly for those already practising, achievement of competencies would have to be demonstrated within a broader integrated career and competency framework, for different specialisms and generalisms. In reality the situation is much less clear. Andrea Bellot is the lead nurse at the Croydon National Health Service (NHS) walk-in centre. In 2002 she had a team of 13 nurses, only five of whom were full time, providing a 365-days a year nurse-led service, and seeing approximately 3,000 patients a

month. The team of nurses are all regarded by Andrea as nurse practitioners. However, without a regulatory framework, as Andrea herself says,
'What is a nurse practitioner?' (Bellot 2002). The team works primarily
with the public entering the centre and clinics with undifferentiated, undiagnosed conditions. To this end Andrea in fact calls her nursing team
primary care practitioners. This may reflect that they are competent, but
their scope of competencies may not entirely fulfil those of nurse practitioner courses accredited by universities, or a professional organisation
such as the Royal College of Nursing (RCN). Andrea reflects on the realities of regulating the role of the nurse practitioner to a specific educational pathway in this extract taken from the interview transcript:

> There's no consistent approach to the higher level of care provision
> within this country at all. There's no consistent approach for training
> and preparation for that higher level of care delivery, and it's insulting
> in a way, to say that somebody who has achieved that higher level of
> practice, even though they haven't been on a nurse practitioner
> course, is not able or entitled to be called a nurse practitioner. I think
> that's crazy. ... We can't afford to send nurses on a two and half year
> nurse practitioner course. There would be nobody left to run the
> service. We are sending nurses because we need to have home grown
> practitioners. I don't believe protecting the nurse practitioner title is
> going to make any difference whatsoever, it's just going to increase
> the status of those people that have that title, purely because they
> have gone through a particular process. I think it's insulting to those
> people who have done it slightly differently, and I think, in a way, if
> you achieve a level of competence that's measurable, it doesn't matter
> how you got there really, as long as you can prove that you're compe-
> tent, and we have particular competencies for our nurses here. They
> have to achieve a certain level of competence. ... I don't think it's fair
> to say that just because you've been through a course that says, you
> are a nurse practitioner, that you should be protected and you should
> have a status above those people that have done it in a slightly differ-
> ent way.
>
> (Bellot 2002)

Andrea's comments reflect the pragmatic approach that nursing is far
from a homogenous occupation and also emphasises the point that undertaking a course does not necessarily make one an expert. Practise within a
continuingly supportive clinical supervision relationship will assist in
achieving this. Nurse practitioners *are* practising and because of the
former lack of regulation for specialist or advanced nursing practice, will
have undertaken a huge variety of modules and courses to enhance their
practice skills. If healthcare increasingly demands the need for nurse practi-

tioners, then too tight a restriction, through regulation to a specific educational preparation, could produce a pseudo-workforce who become Nurse Practitioners under another name.

It is of value to reflect back on British nursing's history, and the attempts to close the profession to the unqualified. The 1919 *Nurse's Registration Act* failed to achieve this, and resulted in not only a variety of supplementary parts to the register, but an ever present army of nursing auxiliaries, generally ignored by the nursing profession, yet providing valuable basic and highly personal care to the public. The 1943 *Nurses' Act* sought to operationalise the 1939 *Interim Report of the Inter-departmental Committee on Nursing Services*. This believed that 'excepting nurses in training, no persons other than state registered nurses or assistant nurses entered on the roll should, habitually and for gain, engage in nursing the sick' (HMSO 1939). By the late 1940s it was estimated there were still some 24,000 nursing auxiliaries, although exact figures were impossible to gain (Abel-Smith 1960). The issue in fact had been influenced by many factors such as the dilution of nursing labour during the war and the close differentials in pay between qualified and unqualified nurses. This made the assistant nurse's two-year training and lack of promotional opportunities at the time, a relatively unattractive proposition. However, it does emphasise the need to consider the workforce itself, and the needs of the service before creating a regulation that may not meet the demands for the skill of the nurse practitioner.

Katrina Maclaine, the course director for the Royal College of Nursing development centre's nurse practitioner degree programme is a part-time nurse practitioner herself. She reflects that with the former lack of any regulatory framework innovation may be encouraged, but questions whether nurses are always aware of the necessary preparation to provide the highest standard of service:

> Students always say we want the title protected, and I also say well, that's fine, but while we're in a grey area, to a certain extent we have the freedom to challenge and push boundaries. If it's laid down in law, it may be very restrictive on what we're currently doing, a bit like the Scope of (Professional) Practice has enabled us to do this. But if it comes in and it's quite rigid, then it could potentially constrict what people are already doing, so it's one of those sort of issues. The trouble is people don't know what they don't know, and what we have is, we have people coming on the course increasingly, who are saying they're working as Nurse Practitioners, they just want the piece of paper. Then they start the course and learn about the many different potential causes of the patient's presenting symptoms and are alarmed to realise that they had been previously working from a very blinkered and potentially unsafe perspective.
>
> (Maclaine 2002)

It would essentially be easier to insist on a specific educational pathway, and be satisfied that because the practitioner had the course they must be forever competent. It is a harder option, yet far more encompassing of the reality of the variety of methods of preparation, to focus on measuring required competencies and to do this on an ongoing developmental basis. The debate will continue as the demand for services grows.

## Clinical supervision

One of the most vital aspects for those involved in running a nurse-led clinic, in terms of maintaining and developing high quality practice, is finding someone who can offer the practitioner effective clinical supervision. Clinical supervision has been described as a formal process of professional support. This aims to enable individual practitioners to develop knowledge and competence and to assume responsibility for their own practice. This ultimately aims to enhance the aforementioned public protection in a variety of clinical situations. Butterworth (1998a) outlines three main goals of the process from Platt-Koch's (1986) work: to expand the therapist's knowledge base, to assist in developing clinical proficiency, to develop autonomy and self-esteem as a professional.

Cutcliffe *et al.* (2001) avoid giving a precise definition of clinical supervision, because they contend that there is no one single way to carry it out. This is due to the subjective nature of the self. We may all have our own personal way of reflecting. Instead, they provide a list of what they term 'assumptions' of what they consider clinical supervision both is and is not. These are contained in Box 2.1. Some of the key elements are the need for the practitioner to feel safe to explore issues and an ability to have nurtured within them the skill of reflection. Reflection is highlighted below because of its advantage in one of the main functions of clinical supervision, which is to move the supervisee through to some form of resolution of the problem or the learning issue they have raised. Highly developed reflective skills are also regarded as an attribute of expertise (Manley and Garbett 2000).

Reflection is in fact a developed skill, if the practitioner is to move beyond merely describing a past event, to making a clear attempt with their supervisor to change and improve his or her practice. It is also of clear value to mention that clinical supervision is an opportunity to reflect on why something went well in practice, and the factors that led to this. Developing a disciplined approach to this also enables reflection-in-action in everyday practice. Reflection and clinical supervision can also be future orientated in terms of exploring possible strategies to address a situation and their consequences.

Implemented correctly this formal process can be invaluable. It allows the opportunity to take time with a colleague who can facilitate the nurse

---

**Box 2.1    Assumptions regarding the role of clinical supervision (after Cutcliffe et al. 2001)**

Clinical supervision is necessarily:

- supportive
- safe, because of clear, negotiated agreements by all parties with regard to the extent and limits of confidentiality
- centred on developing best practice for service users
- brave, because practitioners are encouraged to talk about the realities of their practice
- a chance to talk about difficult areas of work in an environment where the person attempts to understand
- an opportunity to ventilate emotion without comeback
- the opportunity to deal with material and issues that practitioners may have been carrying for many years (the chance to talk about issues which cannot easily be talked about elsewhere and which may have been previously unexplored)
- not to be confused with or amalgamated with managerial supervision
- not to be confused with or amalgamated with personal therapy/counselling
- regular
- protected time
- offered equally to all practitioners
- involving a committed relationship from both parties
- separate and distinct from preceptorship or mentorship
- a facilitative relationship
- challenging
- an invitation to be self-monitoring and self-accountable
- at times hard work and at others enjoyable
- involving developing of reflective skills and becoming a reflective practitioner
- an activity that continues throughout one's working life

---

to explore and articulate the range of evidence underpinning his or her practice, to consider the consequences of their action and develop new practice insights. In addition, it offers the chance to pick apart decision-making and the values inherent in practice. Achieving clinical supervision is much easier said than done, because many nurses in nurse-led clinics work in isolation, often in small teams and frequently have large demands on their time. However, although there may be a feeling of isolation in the role, the nurse does not necessarily have to go outside of the unit, practice or hospital to find a supervisor. The process of clinical supervision begins from within the practitioner, with a supervisor guiding this process.

Therefore searching for someone who is in the same or a similar role is not necessarily a prerequisite.

Figures are hard to gain, but it does appear the uptake of clinical supervision in nursing generally has been patchy. Anecdotally, The Royal Berkshire Hospital and Battle Hospitals NHS Trust suggested an uptake of only 10 per cent in their nursing staff after a six-year programme, while Wandsworth Primary Care Trust offer figures of only 100 actively involved, from 1,300 staff (Cole 2002). The reasons may be multifactorial and include a misunderstanding of the role, process and its benefits, together with a paucity of appropriately prepared staff to offer supervision and their time. These reasons are only suggestions. The RCN for example, has developed UK-wide standards to enable practitioners to become accredited as skilled facilitators/clinical supervisors at three different levels, thus enabling recognition of these valuable skills as well as transferability across the UK (see www.rcn.org.uk/pd).

It is therefore encouraged here that as an important early priority, the nurse needs to take steps to actively put herself/himself into a supervisory relationship. This is often a peer colleague, but it does not have to be someone of the same discipline. Kim Manley is head of practice development at The Royal College of Nursing. Her role, with her team, involves working with organisations to collaboratively develop and implement practice development strategies which are evidence based and patient focussed. As this also includes developing organisation-wide evaluation strategies, this in addition involves researching the subsequent effects on practice. Kim suggests that it can be useful if the clinical supervisor is not in the same nursing specialism, as they can ask what she terms as 'naïve questions' which challenge what we as nurses do (Manley 2002). This also helps us to become aware of our assumptions and the things we take for granted in our everyday practice. The key attribute is someone who the nurse considers will be supportive, and has the confidence to challenge the nurse's practice in a constructive and ultimately developmental way over a continuous period of time. This is together with the two sides' ability to form a trusting relationship.

There appears to be a broad agreement that because of the issue of being willing to share and explore experiences, clinical supervision should be voluntary, but always within collaboratively agreed ground rules. This will inevitably reduce the numbers who participate (Cole 2002). However, Manley (2001) argues from her research, that formal systems of critique and challenge within organisations and teams, such as clinical supervision and action learning, is an attribute of an effective workplace. Developing such systems and skills may therefore be an essential early priority.

For clinical supervision to be effective, there is a need to put aside a regular period of undisturbed time to review particular events, patient encounters or perceived deficits in knowledge. There is a need for the nurse and clinical supervisor to consider beforehand what will be discussed and reviewed during their formal times together. The concept of reflection discussed below and the use of reflective models can help the nurse to tease apart the various elements, which made up the event being discussed. For clinical supervision to be as effective as possible, a suggestion is made here to record salient points of what has been discussed in the nurse's personal portfolio. This is together with the action that is to be planned to address these, such as the need perhaps to sit in with another colleague and observe their assessment skills, to review specific guidelines, to address a learning deficit or indeed any actions in order to maintain what went well. An agreed time needs to be put aside to review the subsequent actions taken, perhaps also by reviewing another event that had similar elements and to see how this differed. This remains a suggestion because of the sometimes personal nature of clinical supervision, and the supervisee may not want any specific notes made. Even so, it is good practice, and would be contracted with the ground rules for the supervisee to take responsibility for documenting their own action points. Subsequent supervision sessions can then start with an update of progress. An action plan can also assist in allowing active steps to be taken to resolve a raised problem.

An alternative to the two-person clinical supervision, is that of group supervision or action learning. Action learning is not discussed within this chapter, but has been defined as 'a continuous process of learning and reflection, supported by colleagues, with an intention of getting things done' (McGill and Beaty 2001: 11). It aims to encourage individuals to use reflection to move an issue forward in practice through group support and self-directed learning. Group members challenge a presenter through questioning directed by a facilitator (Kirrane 2001). The latter author, together with McGill and Beaty (2001), Rayner *et al.* (2002) and Weinstein (1999), provide a useful analysis and practical assistance in this technique. Cole (2002) reports positively on an eight-person clinical supervision group. The advantages are that when a problem is raised by a member of the group and explored, there is a small team who can help offer solutions to the problem, once the presenter has exhausted their own ideas first.

Inevitably the issue of group dynamics enter this form of clinical supervision. Some staff will prefer this method, others will not want to discuss issues they may well have explored if it were a one-to-one situation. If the philosophy of clinical supervision is followed, such options need to be discussed with the team, even though the attraction of a group approach may be that time and staff availability offers a limited possibility of an individual supervisory route. It's worth highlighting that there is evidence that sessions do take much longer when there is a group (Butterworth 1998b), suggesting the issue of making time to meet many people's needs. Normally groups would need to be at least two to three hours once per month, compared with the one-hour session for one-to-one supervision.

## Beginning the process of clinical supervision

Parsons (2000) emphasises the importance of education programmes, often in-house, to equip staff to begin the process of clinical supervision. She advocates the need to address a number of questions and processes within such programmes. These include:

- exploring conceptions of clinical supervision;
- practising holding truly reflective conversations;
- discussing how to move clinical supervision forward;
- discussing how to keep it going – sustainability;
- discussing how we know if it is working – evaluation.

This text can only introduce the concepts of clinical supervision within the wider issues of the nurse-led clinic. A review of texts such as Bassett (1999), Butterworth et al. (1998) and Ghaye and Lillyman (2000) in which Parsons contributes, offer practical assistance in preparing for the implementation of clinical supervision, practising reflective conversations, as well as issues such as evaluation.

As highlighted above, it's vitally important to review with a group or individual, what clinical supervision is. This can often be seen as part of the contracting process. This is regarded as the period before supervision begins when the supervisee(s) and supervisor meet to agree how the process will work for them. This will include issues such as the frequency of meetings, what supervision aims to achieve, the role or responsibilities of the parties involved, the area of confidentiality and how evaluation of the process will be carried out. This may all be agreed in writing and can be kept in the nurse's personal portfolio.

Clinical supervision emerges primarily as a practice-led activity, and not as control or interference in professional autonomy (Butterworth 1998a). Clear guidelines, structure and ground-rules also prevent the group dissolving into a general discussion, although Cole (2002) reports this 'off loading' aspect is valued greatly by staff. It is protected time and not an opportunity for formal teaching or a chance for management to impart new information.

Ground rules need to be set at the start. By their nature these should emerge from the group, but suggestions can be made regarding issues of confidentiality, respecting each others' view points, not offering solutions to members' problems before they have been allowed to explore these themselves, commitment to attendance and so forth. These can be placed on a flip chart and typed up at a later date for group members.

One of the advantages of good clinical supervision is in meeting the ever present practice theory gap. Although not true of all universities, as many are taking steps to develop practice development strategies between themselves and their purchasers, there is always the argument that courses only raise awareness in those who attend. Despite techniques in teaching such as practice based assignments, it often remains unclear whether the money spent does actually result in practice being altered for the better. There can be many reasons why a change of practice may not ultimately occur, either in the nurses running the nurse-led clinic, or in the wider team. Kim Manley highlights two of these reasons. The first is that the practitioner may be unaware of how to achieve sustainable change, and second the system or organisation itself may create barriers which the practitioner may need continuous support and challenge to address (Manley 2002). Clinical supervision can be useful in addressing the issues of why the practitioner finds it difficult to instigate a change. It may also help them to reflect on the factors inherent in the system which are hindering a patient-centred change. As Kim highlights, nurse-led clinics are changing the system, but they are coming up against barriers, and so the question is how can higher education institutions such as universities, and learning methods such as clinical supervision, assist in enabling practitioners to develop the skills necessary to continuously break down resistance to effective change (Manley 2002). Butterworth (1998b) identifies such organisational and management issues as one of the primary areas that were addressed during clinical supervision sessions in a twenty-three site research project in England and Scotland. Such issues dealt with through the learning experiences offered by clinical supervision were instrumental in making positive changes for the organisation. However, on occasion it can just raise an issue that both supervisor and supervisee feel helpless within (Butterwoth 1998b), and that reality perhaps needs to be recognised. Manley therefore argues for the need to balance such feelings of helplessness with leadership/facilitation skills that enable 'a vision of what is possible' to be articulated (Manley 2001). In addition, the use of an external supervisor to the organisation may assist in such a situation, and allow the nurse to feel safe to express and explore issues.

As in all nursing practice, there is a need for evidence that clinical supervision does ultimately improve patient care and services. It is important to consider this, rather than following the traditional line of seizing upon what seems a logical idea. At present it remains controversial whether there is explicit evidence that clinical supervision leads directly to an improvement in quality care. However, Manley and her colleagues have demonstrated the impact of clinical supervision and similar processes on developing a culture of effectiveness – one that is patient-centred and evidence-based, and constantly responding and adapting to a changing context (Manley 2001). A paucity of evidences does not mean the process is ineffective, it is a prompt for further study into its use. Butterworth (1998b) analysed the use of clinical supervision over an eighteen-month period at three time points. Results primarily focussed on benefits to the staff, which were reported as positive. Tentative suggestions can be made that this ultimately improves patient care, but it is this particular area where further research is needed.

Butterworth (1998b) could conclude that in the period under study the control group which did not receive clinical supervision/mentorship showed evidence of increased emotional exhaustion and depersonalisation (through the *Minnesota Job Satisfaction Scale*). After the group received clinical supervision these factors stabilised and sometimes decreased. In supervisors who did not receive clinical supervision themselves, there was a trend towards increased psychological distress.

As a framework to consider evaluation, Butterworth (1998b) suggests three areas to link clinical supervision to clinical outcomes. First is *the normative component*, which addresses organisational and quality control issues. This may be seen through measurements such as clinical audit, staff sickness levels, and staff and patient satisfaction scales. *The restorative component* addresses support for professionals working with stress and distress. This may be seen through a variety of reputable survey instruments. Maslach and Jackson (1986) and Brown *et al.* (1995) are offered as examples. Finally, *the formative component* of developing skills. This may be seen through educational audits which are sensitive to specific clinical skills. These three areas are also useful in providing a direction for a more holistic approach to clinical supervision within the sessions themselves. There are staff both in practice and academia whose primary role is in research and audit. It is of value to link to Trust or University teams that deal with these aspects to gain both advice and support, if the effects of clinical supervision are to be measured. This can be an enlightening and developmental process for all.

Clearly it can be argued that offering staff the chance to reflect and problem solve a situation with another experienced person or team, is likely to have an intrinsic value. It is important for this to be done with another because of the danger of self-delusion. It may also assist in meeting the Government's clinical governance requirements and can be discussed or presented within that framework. By definition, clinical governance is a system through which NHS organisations are accountable for continuously improving the quality of their services and safeguarding high standards of care. This is achieved through creating an environment in which excellence in clinical care will flourish (Scally and Donaldson 1998). The ethos can also be applied to non-NHS organisations.

The role of clinical supervision is obviously not one that can be taken lightly. Of value is creating an open dialogue with the local university provider to consider the most appropriate method of preparing staff for the role, and importantly to allow effective continued development of this skill within the practice area, beyond a one-off course.

Gaining protected time for clinical supervision or any form of staff professional development can be an inflammatory issue with the constant need to meet service requirements. Andrea Bellot highlights that her walk-in centre is closed for three hours each week to allow for team education and the exploration of relevant issues. Service wise, it is not a popular move, but if there is an emergency patients will be seen or advised to come back in a short while. This is much the same as a GP service may offer with their appointment system, but it does allow the team much valued time together. The first hour is assigned to debriefing the team of any Trust wide or services developments. The second hour provides formal teaching, from within the team or from an outside speaker, and the final hour is assigned to looking at perhaps a patient's notes, a new drug, a Patient Group Direction (PGD) or a specific condition.

It is easy to outline what can be achieved, but time and the skill mix of the team can often mitigate against effective clinical supervision. However, there is a clear need for those in nurse-led clinics to consider how clinical supervision can be used as a formal structure, beyond an informal approach of sharing ideas in the coffee room, or providing articles to read. In addition, finding the right person to offer the supervision may mean that no one person can meet all the desired needs. It is probably more important to consider what are the desired outcomes of the supervision. This may mean that if the issue is to enhance clinical practice, one person may be chosen, while another is sought for issues of management or counselling skills. There are many developing and unique roles described in this book under the umbrella of the nurse-led clinic. It may be that the person feels, whether a nurse practitioner, practice nurse, nurse consultant and so forth, that only a person in the same role can understand the intricacies and professional challenges of that role. This inevitably makes achieving effective clinical supervision in potentially isolating roles quite difficult, but not impossible.

## Reflective practice

Reflection, both *in* and *on practice*, has been actively encouraged within nursing and curricula development for a number of years. Reflection in practice generally refers to the process where the practitioner recognises a new situation and considers aspects of problem solving while still present in the work or clinical area. Reflection-on-action is a retrospective analysis to consider the knowledge used in a practice situation and the areas of personal knowledge or skill deficit. The reflective practitioner may speculate how the situation might have been handled differently and what other knowledge would have helped in the situation (Schon 1987).

Donald Schon is regarded as having a significant influence on reflection within nursing practice. His celebrated text *The Reflective Practitioner* (Schon 1991) originally published in 1983, was not the first to discuss reflection, but it has been one of the most influential. Schon discussed the issue of 'technical rationality' (Schon 1991: 21–69). This refers to professionals making decisions and solving problems primarily through the application of scientific theory and technique. This he charts historically as developing and accompanying the decline in religion, superstition and mysticism, with ideas founded increasingly on positivistic science. As Hannigan (2001) describes in his discussion on the strengths and weaknesses of reflection, Schon argues that technical rationality cannot account for all that professionals do. The problems they solve are rarely abstract or clear cut. Problems occur in particular settings and solutions are therefore found only in the specific contexts in which problems are framed (Hannigan 2001). For Schon, reflection is a way for practitioners to bridge the practice-theory gap, with the skill having the ability to uncover knowledge in and on action. Practitioners have tacit 'knowing in action' (Schon 1987: 25; Schon 1991: 49). This is the knowledge practitioners possess, but may not be entirely aware of. It is implicit, and reflection can assist the practitioner to articulate what they know and how they have come to know it. Once explicit, it can be used to change and enhance practice.

Schon reinforced his view through the discussion of an area he termed as 'swampy lowland'. This he contrasted to the area of context-free, high, hard ground, where the focus is on the development of theoretical knowledge rather than its use. In the swampy lowland, situations are confusing and incapable of technical solution (Schon 1991: 42). Reflection can therefore aid in examining care provided and assist in problem solving. It has to be seen as a structured process of analysing a particular event or events from or in practice. The reflective process is not merely a general discussion regarding an event, or reassuring a clinical supervisor that everything was fine. There is a need to tease out the elements which made it a positive, negative or just an ordinary everyday experience for both practitioner and patient. This is in addition to considering those areas which need to be enhanced through learning to ultimately improve patient care, when a similar or the same situation is met again. It is this ability to identify specifically what happened, which can also allow the clinical supervisor to enable the practitioner to reinforce their own skills or assist the practitioner to see for themselves where learning deficits still lie.

Often reflection is presented in a cycle, which suggests it is an ongoing process in practice. This also suggests that the circle needs to be closed by taking assertive action to meet the learning deficits. Page and Meerabeau (2000) refer to this as 'closing the loop'. Such learning needs can be planned as part of clinical supervision, and reviewed at a later date.

Reflection has therefore often been seen as synonymous with clinical supervision, because of its perceived value in sharing an experience with a knowledgeable mentor to enhance practice. However, it is a skill which can be an ongoing part of personal and individual practice. Of the variety of tools available to offer structure to the process, which have included Driscoll (1994), Gibbs (1988) and Johns (1995); Taylor (2001) presents a

---

**Box 2.2    Reflective questions (after Taylor 2001: 56)**

What went well?
Why did it go well?
Where did it happen?
Who was involved?
How were they involved?
How were you involved?
What did you do?
What were the consequences for yourself and others?
Why did you do what you did?
What were you thinking at the time?
What do you think about it now?

---

useful set of initial questions to begin the process, for those who may not be familiar with the technique.

As Taylor (2001) emphasises, the nurse may not be able to bring all of his/her knowledge to the surface in response to this reflector. However, the skill does generally develop and the nurse becomes more used to freer thinking, and the ability to connect thoughts to reach fresh insights about personal practice. It is important to state that for reflection to be as effective as possible, it is a skill that needs to be practised and guided by the tools that are now available to enhance its effectiveness. Particularly if the nurse and the person offering clinical supervision are inexperienced in reflection, taking the time to choose an event and apply the model prior to meeting, can enhance the time together, beyond a pleasant chat about a key clinical encounter. Reflection is highly personal and it's a technique which requires that an honest and trusted relationship between the practitioner and their clinical supervisor is formed and based around negotiated ground rules and ongoing evaluation. It can be a cathartic experience that lays bear practice issues that need improving, as well as areas that need maintaining.

### The reflexive practitioner

It is of value to highlight at this point the idea of the 'reflexive practitioner', because this links both to reflection-in-action and is of value within the role of clinical supervision. Rolfe (1997) argues that the expert or reflexive practitioner makes practice seem simple and effortless because they are 'functioning on autopilot'. There is the unconscious drawing on his/her repertoire of paradigm cases (Rolfe 1997: 96). The reflexive practitioner utilises reflection-*in*-action rather than retrospectively reflecting. He or she utilises on the spot experimenting, with the generation of informal theory and the testing of hypotheses in the practice situation. The reflexive practitioner needs to be acutely aware of the clinical situation they are in. In performing a skill every move, every decision is thought about, relating these to *this* patient in *this* situation. They would be learning from their performance, thinking about how it could be done differently and constructing an informal theory regarding how to problem solve or address the situation. This is based on *this* informal knowledge, but also on past paradigm cases and formal, research based theory.

A hypothesis is tested by making a clinical intervention. There is then reflection on the transformed clinical situation, with actions modified in the here and now and added to personal knowledge. This all requires mindful attention with reflective practice occurring in vivo (Rolfe 1997). Therefore for clinical supervision to assist in enhancing practice, it is useful to reflect on reflection-in-action. This assists in reviewing the above actions and issues to consider what was learnt and to recognise that in a similar encountered situation this new knowledge can be considered and a hypothesis once more tested.

### Does reflection work?

It remains clear that currently there is a large amount of literature regarding the apparent benefits and advantages of reflection, yet there remains a paucity of empirical research into the clinical outcomes (nursing or patient) consequent to reflective practice (Paget 2001). Paget (2001) explored whether 200 nurses from both pre- and post-registered undergraduate courses, a post-registered diploma module and a post-registered Masters in nursing course, perceived any change in their clinical practice, which could be attributed to reflection. A small number were accessed via focus groups, while postal questionnaires were sent to all 200. Seventy-two questionnaires were returned. Telephone interviews occurred with a further 10 of those who returned the questionnaires. The nurses generally valued the formal use of reflection within their studies, while 78 per cent believed that significant, specific change had taken place (Paget 2001). This was generally seen as long lasting.

Such results are encouraging, but the need to measure change in practice remains clear. However, if staff feel the process is of value to their practice, this can be *anticipated* as beneficial to patient care, even if only making explicit areas that warrant personal or organisational change. This may then be linked to an action plan to initiate or begin the process of change. It is this final step that appears the most problematic, the 'closing of the loop' to ensure effective and beneficial change from reflection. Rolfe (2002) argues that experiential knowledge from reflection-on-action now finds itself at the bottom of the hierarchy of evidence on which to base practice. This is because of the domination of the evidence-based paradigm. A paradigm is concerned with how a discipline organises and manages its knowledge base. In a thought provoking paper Rolfe (2002) considers how we can move more towards a reflective paradigm. This would involve a variety of steps, including the need for the paradigm to focus primarily on the development of practice rather than theory. Rolfe argues that currently, the development of nursing practice is seen as a secondary goal of research, achieved through the application of research-based knowledge to clinical settings (Rolfe 2002).

Johns (1999) reflects on the organisation or culture, which limits the realisation of reflection. He considers the results of reflection being placed within a culture that has historically limited its realisation, and where it can become compromised in achieving both empowering and emancipatory intent (Johns 1999). Where the guide or supervisor to reflection is stained by the brush of the organisation, then the guide may wittingly or unwittingly act in such ways to reinforce organisational values (Johns 1999). Fostering such a change is a difficult issue, with Page and Meerabeau (2000) suggesting the need to include the planning and management of change as an integral part of the reflective cycle. One of the values of nurse-led clinics and services, is that they are breaking new ground, and re-establishing the practice boundaries. With planning, is the opportunity to consider the issue of practices we sometimes take for granted such as reflection, and how we can close that loop as a team, or even disregard the technique as valuable to practice, through a continued inability to create such closure.

## The use of competencies within the nurse-led clinic

The current use of competencies appears to pervade all nursing life. Their clear value is in breaking apart a role or job into small bite size chunks that can be both measured and utilised to develop appropriate professional development. The term competency was described by the UKCC in 1999 as describing the skills and ability to practise safely and effectively without the need for direct supervision (UKCC 1999). Competencies can therefore be seen as statements or a claim pertaining to skills, tasks or roles that are carried out effectively.

There is often some confusion between competencies, outcomes and standards, because all are used within practice. Even within the single terms there can be differing interpretation, as Manley and Garbett (2000) demonstrate when examining competency (Manley and Garbett 2000: 349). There is to a degree some overlap between the above terms, because if you are competent in a skill inevitably the standard of your practice will rise. However, there is also the issue of equity, that a nurse may be competent in an area, but the actual practice itself may not be at the higher standard of perhaps another colleague. For example, if the nurse were competent in taking a clinical history, but appeared disinterested, was constantly answering the telephone during the assessment, allowed colleagues to come in and out of the clinical room and so forth, they may be deemed by some as competent in gaining the clinical history, but the standard of that consultation was low. Standards therefore provide benchmarks, which ensure that the competency is fulfilled to a specific quality level.

An example of a set of standards would be those within one of the last documents published by the UKCC, for determining a higher level of practice. These fell within seven categories, and the breakdown within each was regarded as the standard or quality of practice that had to be met for the nurse to be considered as functioning at that higher level. By their own definition a standard is 'a collection of specific outcome statements against which a practitioner's performance can be assessed with validity and reliability' (UKCC 2002: 9). The latter two terms are essentially linked to the skill of research. Validity relates to whether the tool used to measure something has captured the essence or truth of what it is supposed to be measuring. Reliability relates to the accuracy of a tool. A measurement tool can be accurate, but it may not be the correct tool for the assessment, therefore it may not be valid. The term 'outcomes' tends to refer to the result of practice rather than the activities or tasks that lead to the result (UKCC 2002).

Competencies are increasingly being used to create criteria to classify or clarify nursing roles. The RCN have been developing through their membership network, an integrated career and competency framework for different specialist groups linked with *Agenda For Change*, the government's proposals to modernise the NHS pay system and conditions of service (DOH 1999). This aims to provide a UK-wide framework for enabling patients to receive the same level of care regardless of where they access that care, for a number of different specialisms. This has been created from developing a common vision about the purpose of the specialism and how this purpose is achieved, using value clarification with as many practitioners as possible UK-wide.

In addition, by teasing out competencies for both general and more specific nursing roles, it can provide an explicit clinical career ladder for which practitioners can progress as well as ultimately linking this to remuneration. The RCN website offers an ongoing update and review of progress in relation to *Agenda for Change*: www.rcn.org.uk. In addition, competencies can be seen again in the RCN's *Domains and Competencies for UK Nurse Practitioner Practice* (RCN 2002). Here a professional organisation had attempted to protect the public and produce an equitable service by stating, in their view, certain competencies that should be measurably achieved for the nurse to be called a nurse practitioner.

There are at present no legal requirements supporting this document, and there is a reliance on individual nurses and employers to adhere to the competency framework if the title is being used. However, they are based on extensive experience from the United States and now the UK, and provide a unifying framework through their core elements for all nurse practitioners. This document also has a set of standards, to ensure that those nurse practitioner courses that are accredited by the RCN are delivered at a measurable level of quality. The question is whether the RCN document is of value to the nurse-led clinic. The answer is simply that they are of clear value to those calling themselves a nurse practitioner, and may offer guidance to others running nurse-led clinics. As discussed throughout this book, nurse-led clinics are currently run by a variety of nurses who beyond registration will have gained differing educational preparation, in varying skills and specialities. Such competencies are of value, but remain specific to the particular role of nurse practitioner.

## How can competencies assist in the nurse-led clinic?

When a nurse-led clinic is developed, a job description will usually be generated. This primarily guides the choice of candidate, and allows applicants to consider whether the post would be correct for their personal aspirations and skills. Occasionally, the role becomes an extension of a nurse's current duties and he or she may help develop the job description. What may invariably be true, is that even if a broad job description is in place at the start, as the nurse-led clinic develops, it may ultimately bear little resemblance to the eventual service offered and the role of the practitioner. Emma Martin runs a nurse-led clinic for male patients with erectile dysfunction linked to cardiovascular disease, at St Thomas' Hospital in London. Emma and consultant nurse for cardiology, Elaine Coady, reflect on the issues of the job description in these extracts taken from their interview transcript (Martin and Coady 2002):

> Emma: The job description wasn't very specific. It talked about setting up a service. It talked about running a clinic. It wasn't very, very specific.
>     Elaine: ... vague enough for you to allow Emma to have the scope to be able to determine how that service was going to evolve, and I think it has evolved over the year, and I think again there's even more scope for it to evolve with Emma's role within that clinic changing as time goes on. So although there may have been a bit of hesitancy to start with, about whether it was nurse led, I think with Emma's experience so far, and how we see the service going, I'm sure it will develop into ... I mean you'll be doing, probably, the physical assessment and the prescribing.

Emma: I would say now, a year on, the clinic's been running from March. ... I would say although there are things that I'm not doing, I'm clear in my own mind the clinic is nurse led, whereas in the beginning, certainly for the first few months, sort of finding my feet, with my medical colleagues, you know, determining what we wanted to be looking at, disagreeing, and finding our way. ... I felt less confident about saying it was nurse led, but now I feel more confident.

This element of an evolving clinic and even determining whether it *is* nurse-led, from the responsibilities, autonomy devoid of strong medical control and specific roles undertaken, lends itself to the required clarity of a competency framework. As highlighted in the section discussing clinical supervision, it is strongly recommended that the nurse running the clinic has a personal education portfolio for his or her own professional development. In this, kept within the clinic, can be the job description and an ongoing plan of development based upon a set of competencies created from the description itself. These need to be specific and measurable and break the role into its smaller parts. This then accompanies any criteria to demonstrate that the competency has been achieved. This is together with an initial 'action plan' identifying how the practitioner intends to learn or enhance the competency. Maggie McCowan, a senior nurse in infection control in Glasgow, was part of a team developing clinically specific competency descriptors. She believes competencies offer a clear message to practitioners about continuing professional development: 'I think you're saying to do this job effectively this is the knowledge you need, this is how you can get it, this is how you could apply it and this is how you could learn from it and reflect on it. It's a live thing, it's not sitting down burning the midnight oil, just reading dusty tomes – it's something you carry with you everyday of your practice' (NBS 2001: 7).

## Assessing clinical competence

The assessment of clinical competence within the nurse-led clinic is likely to occur in a variety of situations. For example, the nurse may be attending a course to learn new skills or to update. In this situation, and provided there is a practice based element, an assessor may come and visit the clinical area to assess the nurse in practice, or a mentor will be chosen by the nurse to assist them in completing this element of the course. Neary (2000) identifies several roles of the assessor to make the process of assessment as fulfilling and valid as possible. Assessors are expected to know the process by which the system of continuous assessment is conducted for those students for whom they are responsible. Their knowledge is gained from:

- attendance, not only at the preparatory course, but also at follow-up sessions;
- adequate familiarisation with the documentation used for the recording of student progress;
- continued professional development.

It is clearly desirable to fulfil all three; it is likely that the first is more of an ideal in a busy team. However, it is the responsibility of the assessor to take time to read the material used for assessment, before undertaking any assessment role, and to have access to the course tutor (telephone contact, e-mail and so forth) so that questions can be easily answered. It is also the responsibility of the tutor to return calls as promptly as possible. 'Professional development' refers in part to the need for attendance at short courses, run for example by the local university regarding mentorship, assessing and teaching in clinical practice. Such material can then be dissipated throughout the team at meetings with appropriate staff. Of clear advantage is for the team to acquire a small selection of articles and/or texts on the skill of assessment, and a variety now exist.

The other area of assessment that has been discussed within this text, is the need to ensure the nurse running the clinic is developing relevant competencies. This is to ensure provision of a measurably appropriate, safe and high standard of service. In addition, is the need for those areas and skills where the nurse claims competence to be up to date and indeed of an appropriate standard for the role. Bellot (2002) highlighted above, a set of competencies for her nurses which ensure a general standard of service for the walk-in centre. The nurse practitioner competencies created by the RCN are of great value in producing core competencies to help ensure this standard approach. As highlighted, for the individual nurse, breaking apart the role undertaken, often with the assistance of the job description, can help create an appropriate teaching plan. This can both assess current competencies on a periodic basis and aid development of those that are new, but required for the role.

There are several issues with assessment that always appear to produce anxiety. One is the time that assessing all these competencies can take, and also the anxiety produced with someone coming in and watching the practitioner with what traditionally is the pen and paper recording technique. Assessment in education however, has evolved into a much wider concept, and now generally takes into account the idea of professional *development* – that is assessment over time.

Once competencies have been identified, it is of value to allow the nurses themselves to consider how competent they feel in the various skills or areas. It may be useful to ask them to consider a scale of 1 to 6, with *no experience* being 1 and 6 being *competent*, to give the manager or the person providing clinical supervision an idea of where they are, both in the competency itself and in the overall job role. The term 'no experience' or 'limited experience' is used, rather than the negative term of 'not competent'. This approach also helps address the need for a partnership in professional development, between those involved in the assessment process.

There is a need to think broadly if the nurse claims competence, as to how this can be measured or demonstrated. One useful method is the creation of a portfolio of evidence. This can be kept within the wider personal education portfolio in a section dedicated to that competency. The evidence can aim to extend over a specific period of time, perhaps a number of weeks or a few months. After this time the evidence collated, can be reviewed and a summary written regarding whether the competency has been achieved, or indeed needs further development before it is carried out without any form of supervision. The portfolio can contain a variety of evidence, with the choice and appropriateness decided between the nurse and the assessor/clinical supervisor. It is important that the practitioner explains how and why the evidence demonstrates that competency has been achieved, rather than just compiling the evidence.

The advantage of a portfolio is that it empowers the nurse to take responsibility for their own professional development. It also has the scope to consider a variety of evidence sources, and importantly, it occurs over time. This latter point helps to avoid the fear of a one-off assessment, particularly through someone watching the nurse, and everything being

---

**Box 2.3   Portfolio evidence of competency attainment/sources of learning (adapted from NBS 2001)**

Assessment – self/other
Supervisor statements
Clinical supervision
Appraisal reports
Case studies
Reports/proposals
Minutes of meetings
Documents
Personal reports
Exams – written/oral
Projects/workbooks
Literature reviews
Essays
Dissertations/theses
Research/audits
Videos/audio tapes
Reflective accounts
Analytical evaluation

focussed on this single time point. Often in skills-based learning on a course, several time points will be chosen for assessment, to allow the skill to be improved and honed before a final value on the achievement of the competency is given. Competencies do have the potential disadvantage of being behaviourally based. This means there is a need to ensure the thought processes, or critical thinking elements are made explicit. This may be achieved through questioning the rationale behind choices made, asking the nurse to verbally break apart the skill, and exploring where the skill may fit into the wider picture of assessment.

Assessment is always problematic, because it is subjective and it may be difficult to clearly state whether the competency has or has not been achieved. Reviewing a small series of assessments over time, can help the assessor make a more realistic decision. In addition, an issue such as unsafe practice may often be clear to all, but realistically it can often be far more subtle. If for example, the nurse were to miss a safety element such as checking the desired name and date on an X-ray, it is of value to ask an open, non-leading question at the end of the assessment to ascertain their knowledge of this. This may be asking if they know of any safety checks they could make at the start of reviewing an X-ray. If this is highlighted, the knowledge is present and this can be reviewed again in practice as the skill is reassessed over the chosen time period. If it is continually missed out, then achievement of the competency has to be questioned.

Figure 2.1 offers one example of how a competency can be identified, the resources planned to learn or update the skill, and an agreement made between the nurse and the assessor or clinical supervisor, regarding how its achievement will be demonstrated.

To some, the overall action plan can be termed as the learning contract. This particular action plan has some areas of interest. It is a measurable competency, there has been a decision regarding how measurement will be achieved, and it is time related. There is a need with a skill such as that identified in Figure 2.1 to be able to demonstrate in practice the competency is being achieved. Therefore, there is the agreement that the clinical supervisor will periodically provide a series of X-rays and the nurse will discuss the findings. The supervisor will then complete a sheet created within the personal education portfolio, identifying the date, type of X-ray shown to the nurse, and a narrative identifying his/her ability to identify the relevant areas. Note also the important element of referring on to another skilled colleague if the nurse considers that the X-ray does not demonstrate the elements that they are competent in identifying. Referring onwards is not a sign of competency achievement, if the elements are present that they should be able to identify, but it helps address the issue of working within a safe personal scope of practice. Of value is the need to discuss, before the assessment, what the assessor is actually looking for. It is both unfair and inappropriate to teach or allow someone to acquire a

| Competency statement | Learning resources | Evidence of achievement | Time frame |
|---|---|---|---|
| 1. Identifies the chest X-ray with no pathology or abnormalities – the 'clinically normal' chest X-ray<br><br>2. Identifies the more common chest X-ray pathologies (initial 10 pathologies identified and agreed with clinical supervisor). Refers findings to appropriate colleague, together with those identified pathologies that cannot be named | Attend university study day reviewing chest X-ray interpretation on 23 February and 21 March. Inform clinical supervisor if the study day is full, to allow further planning<br><br>Dedicated personal study from text 'Chest X-ray in practice' – chosen text<br><br>Review at each clinical supervision session two X-rays selected blindly by clinical supervisor from the chosen 10<br><br>Consider potential causes of identified pathologies with clinical supervisor | Pass associated assessment on chest X-ray study day and store this in portfolio<br><br>Correctly identify over three consecutive assessment periods 3 chest X-rays chosen at random by clinical supervisor from the agreed 10. This will include the 'normal' chest X-ray<br><br>Discuss relevant referrals to appropriate colleague(s)<br><br>Correctly identify the more common potential causes of the identified pathologies<br><br>Clinical supervisor to record date, pathology and practitioner's assessment, together with supportive feedback within the portfolio | Twelve weeks agreed for assessment process (open to review) |

| Competency statement | Time 1 | Time 2 | Time 3 |
|---|---|---|---|
| Assessor's signature/date | | | |
| Student/nurse's signature/date | | | |

*Figure 2.1* Action plan for competency achievement.

skill, and then not discuss what elements are being reviewed for the assessment. These can be noted on the action plan, or agreed on the assessment sheet that the assessor will use.

Some assessment sheets on courses and in practice may in fact be very brief, but clear discussion regarding areas to be noted should be shared. For many it is a leap of faith to move away from more traditional methods of assessment, perhaps examinations, essays and one-off assessments by staff from higher education. However, there is a need to consider realistically the best way of demonstrating competence, and often it is through assessing over time, with someone who is clinically competent, but with whom the nurse is comfortable and has built up a rapport. It is also important to discuss the pathway to follow if the competency is clearly not being achieved, and to offer support, guidance and a further plan of action.

## Developing methods of education provision

As a concluding section to this chapter, it is of value to clarify some of the alternative methods of education provision that may effect the development of the nurse-led clinic. The reader can then consider how the various methods may fit into the aspirations of their own nurse-led clinic or service. Distance learning has been in place for many years. This is essentially removing the boundaries of the classroom environment, to allow learning to occur at a time and place more suited to the student. It can appeal to two student groups, those who do not wish to study with other people, and those who prefer traditional study, but simply cannot do it due to work and family responsibilities (Pearce 2001). Universities and institutions that run accredited distance learning courses now provide a wide variety of material through printed, video, DVD, audio and computer based sources. These allow interaction with the issues being discussed by specific exercises, activities and reflections.

Courses still run to a specific time frame, with the usual rigour of any university course. Courses or modules will start at specific points in the year and will end at a specific time, as with courses delivered with a classroom basis. Local tutors are available to discuss issues, and summer schools or study days outside of the usual working hours, perhaps at the weekend, do offer the opportunity to mix and share ideas with fellow students. Distance learning does take a particular type of student, who is disciplined with their time. It has been argued that these elements of self-direction and self-responsibility empower nurses to function more autonomously and confidently within their clinical environment (Kenworthy and Dearnley 2001). Research continues regarding the actual impact of such learning modalities on the individual and their ability to deliver high quality care (Kenworthy and Dearnley 2001). It is worth remembering that with distance learning the outcomes still have to be achieved and submitted to a set time frame.

Course work commitments can quickly build up if time management skills are not addressed at an early stage. In addition, with this form of course delivery and with work based learning discussed below, there is the issue of how a unified and shared expansion of roles for the nurse-led clinic and nurse practitioners can be forged if learners work in isolation. There is still a great value in meeting with colleagues regularly to share ideas and clarify roles, particularly for those such as the nurse practitioner where regulation is a more recent concept. Dowd (2000) provides a useful insight into some of the potential benefits, but also disadvantages, of the technological advances in knowledge delivery.

Work-based learning is not a new concept. Work placements have a long history in higher education, particularly with their use as part of sandwich courses (Duckenfield and Stirner 1992; Gray 2001). Work-based learning has been defined as learning at higher education level derived from undertaking paid or unpaid work (Garnett 1997). It can also be defined as clinical supervision and action learning where the focus is on work-based issues leading to professional accreditation, as well as optional academic accreditation. Gray (2001) emphasises it is the means through which a discipline is delivered and not the discipline itself. Generally, it is learning through work linked to an accredited programme of study. It includes learning for work, such as through work placements; learning at work, perhaps through in-house training programmes; and learning through work, linked to formally accredited further or higher education.

It therefore has quite a wide remit, but aims to make the education of the student far more relevant to the role they actually perform. It further attempts to bring the practice-theory gap together. It may also become of greater use in nursing, as the ability to release students from the workplace becomes more and more difficult. However, as can already be seen, it is not by any means a transfer of the classroom to the workplace. It requires a philosophical shift in learning, from the more traditional ways of thinking of course delivery. The student is highly pro-active in this, rather than accepting a set of learning objectives they must achieve. In addition, it requires a tripartite approach from the academic supervisor, the employer and the student (Parish 2001). Approaches can also incorporate an element where prior learning is accredited (Parish 2001). Certain courses are offered completely in this format, others have particular elements delivered through work-based learning, together with taught modules.

Gray (2001) centres work-based learning around reflection on work practices, and not merely acquiring knowledge and a set of technical skills. It is based upon learning arising from action and problem solving within a working environment, centred around chosen live projects and challenges to individuals and organisations. The frameworks designed for such courses aim to have the rigour of those delivered in other formats. Learning outcomes for the particular module will have to be achieved within chosen, negotiated projects and agreed personal learning objectives. It needs to be of benefit to the workplace as well as to the student. Once again the demonstration of evidence will be agreed in the tripartite relationship to meet the requirements of the awarded credits. These can also be dictated by the agreed assessment method for a specific module's learning outcomes. For example, it may be the requirement of the module that a work-based written assignment of 4,000 words will be required for the student to reflect on the process of their chosen project of setting up a new health promotion service for patients. Self-assessment by students also plays an important role in their contribution to this particular type of learning. This can assist in evaluating the project and develop the student's awareness of their own abilities and needs within a role. This links to the issue of reflection discussed above.

In conclusion, this chapter has addressed some of the educational issues that can affect the nurse-led clinic. The need for a supervisory relationship to enhance practice is strongly recommended. The use of competency frameworks is suggested as a method of teasing apart the elements of a role, and creating an appropriate education programme for professional development. Techniques, such as clinical supervision and reflection, may aid competent and developing practice, but their effectiveness needs to be continually evaluated. Pressure on time within the clinics, means that the purchase of education, or its planning with higher education institutions, may need to consider a variety of delivery methods. This chapter has aimed to evaluate some of these methods to empower those involved in purchasing.

## References

Abel-Smith, B. (1960) *A History of the Nursing Profession*, London: Heinemann, pp. 238.

Bassett, C. (ed.) (1999) *Clinical Supervision: A Guide for Implementation*, London: Nursing Times Books.

Bellot, A. (2002) Interview conducted with Andrea Bellot, Lead Nurse at the NHS Walk-in Centre, Croydon, 13 March.

Brown, D., Leary, J., Carson, J., Bartlett, H. and Fagin, L. (1995) 'Stress and the community mental health nurse: the development of a measure', *Journal of Psychiatric and Mental Health Nursing* 2, 1–5.

Butterworth, T. (1998a) 'Clinical supervision as an emerging idea in nursing', in Butterworth, T., Faugier, J. and Burnard, P. (eds) *Clinical Supervision and Mentorship in Nursing*, 2nd edn, Cheltenham: Stanley Thornes Ltd, pp. 1–18.

Butterworth, T. (1998b) 'Evaluation research in clinical supervision: a case example', in Butterworth, T., Faugier, J. and Burnard, P. (eds) *Clinical Supervision and Mentorship in Nursing*, 2nd edn, Cheltenham: Stanley Thornes Ltd, pp. 221–231.

Butterworth, T., Faugier, J. and Burnard, P. (eds) (1998) *Clinical Supervision and Mentorship in Nursing*, 2nd edn, Cheltenham: Stanley Thornes Ltd.

Cole, A. (2002) 'Someone to watch over you', *Nursing Times* 98(23), 22–24.

Cox, C.L. (2001) 'Advanced Nurse Practitioners and Physician Assistants: what is the difference? Comparing the USA and UK', *Hospital Medicine* 62(3), 169–171.

Cox, C.L. (2002) Interview conducted with Professor Carol Cox, Professor of Advanced Clinical Practice, St Bartholomew School of Nursing and Midwifery, City University, London, 15 July.

Cutcliffe, J.R., Butterworth, T. and Proctor, B. (2001) 'Introduction: fundamental themes in clinical supervision: national and international perspectives of education, policy, research and practice', in Cutcliffe, J.R., Butterworth, T. and Proctor, B. (eds) *Fundamental Themes in Clinical Supervision*, London: Routledge, pp. 1–5.

Department of Health (1999) *Agenda for Change: Modernising the NHS Pay System*, London: DOH.

Dowd, C. (2000) 'Virtual learning', *Nursing Management* 7(7), 22–27.

Driscoll, J. (1994) 'Reflective practice for practise', *Senior Nurse* 13(7), 47–50.

Duckenfield, M. and Stirner, P. (1992) *Higher Education Developments: Learning Through Work. The Integration of Work-Based Learning Within Academic Programmes in Higher Education*, Sheffield: Employment Department Group.

Garnett, J. (1997) 'Quality assurance in work-based learning', in UACE Work-Based Learning Network Conference.

Ghaye, T. and Lillyman, S. (eds) (2000) *Effective Clinical Supervision: The Role of Reflection*, Salisbury, Wilts: Quay Books.

Gibbs, G. (1988) *Learning by Doing. A Guide to Teaching and Learning Methods*, Oxford: Further Education Unit, Oxford Polytechnic. Cited also in Palmer, A., Burns, S. and Bulman, C. (eds) (1994) *Reflective Practice in Nursing: The Growth of the Professional Practitioner*, Oxford: Blackwell Science.

Gray, D. (2001) 'Learning and Teaching Support Network Generic Centre: Assessment series No. 11', *A Briefing on Work-based Learning*, York: LTSN.

Greenhalgh & Co. Ltd (1994) *The Interface Between Junior Doctors and Nurses: A Research Study for the Department of Health*, Vol. 1, report. Cheshire: Greenhalgh & Co. Ltd.

Hannigan, B. (2001) 'A discussion of the strengths and weaknesses of "reflection" in nursing practice and education', *Journal of Clinical Nursing* 10, 278–283.

HMSO (1939) *The Inter-departmental Committee on Nursing Services: Interim Report*, Ministry of Health and Board of Education, London: HMSO, pp. 68, para. 165.

Johns, C. (1995) 'Framing learning through reflection with Carper's Fundamental Ways of Knowing in Nursing', *Journal of Advanced Nursing* 22, 226–234.

Johns, C. (1999) 'Reflection as empowerment?', *Nursing Inquiry* 6, 241–249.

Kenworthy, D. and Dearnley, C. (2001) 'Achieving lifelong learning in nursing', *Professional Nurse* 16(6), 1162–1164.

Kirrane, C. (2001) 'Using action learning in reflective practice', *Professional Nurse* 16(5), 1102–1105.

Maclaine, K. (2002) Interview conducted with Katrina Maclaine, Course Director, Nurse Practitioner BSc (Hons) Nurse Practitioner (Primary Health Care) Degree Programme, Royal College of Nursing Development Centre, London South Bank University, 6 March. Interview amended with Katrina Maclaine 3 February 2003.

Manley, K. (1996) 'Advanced practice is not about medicalising nursing roles', *Nursing in Critical Care* 1(2), 3–4 (editorial).

Manley, K. (2001) *Consultant Nurse: Concept, Processes, Outcomes*, Manchester/London: University of Manchester/RCN Institute. Unpublished PhD Thesis.

Manley, K. (2002) Interview conducted with Kim Manley, Head of Practice Development, Royal College of Nursing Headquarters, London, 18 January.

Manley, K. and Garbett, R. (2000) 'Paying Peter and Paul: reconciling concepts of expertise with competency for a clinical career structure', *Journal of Clinical Nursing* 9, 347–359.

Martin, E. and Coady, E. (2002) Focus group interview with nurse Emma Martin and Nurse Consultant, Elaine Coady at St Thomas' Hospital, London, 15 January.

Maslach, C. and Jackson, S. (1986) *Maslach Burnout Inventory*, California: Consulting Psychologists Press.

McGill, I. and Beaty, L. (2001) *Action Learning*, revised 2nd edn, London: Kogan Page Ltd.

NBS (2001) *The Experience of Developing Clinical Competency Descriptors: Some Shared Views*, Scotland: National Board for Nursing, Midwifery and Health Visiting for Scotland.

Neary, M. (2000) *Teaching, Assessing and Evaluation for Clinical Competence: A Practical Guide for Practitioners and Teachers*, Cheltenham: Stanley Thornes Ltd.

Nursing and Midwifery Council (2003) *NMC confirms details of new three-part register*, NMC press statement 7 March. www.nmc-uk.org.

Page, S. and Meerabeau, L. (2000) 'Achieving change through reflective practice: closing the loop', *Nurse Education Today* 20, 365–372.

Paget, T. (2001) 'Reflective practice and clinical outcomes: practitioner's views on how reflective practice has influenced their clinical practice', *Journal of Clinical Nursing* 10, 204–214.

Parish, C. (2001) 'Learn while you work', *Nursing Standard* 26(16), 16–17.

Parsons, G. (2000) 'Some reflections on the implementation of clinical supervision', in Ghaye, T. and Lillyman, S. (eds) *Effective Clinical Supervision: The Role of Reflection*, Salisbury, Wilts: Quay Books.

Pearce, L. (2001) 'Distant horizons', *Nursing Standard* 26(16), 16–17.

Platt-Koch, L.M. (1986) 'Clinical supervision for psychiatric nurses', *Journal of Psycho-Social Nursing* 26(1), 7–15.

Rayner, D., Chisholm, H. and Appleby, H. (2002) 'Developing leadership through action learning', *Nursing Standard* 16(29), 37–39.

Rolfe, G. (1997) 'Beyond expertise: theory, practice and the reflexive practitioner', *Journal of Clinical Nursing* 6, 93–97.

Rolfe, G. (2002) 'Reflective practice: where now?', *Nurse Education in Practice* 2, 21–29.

Royal College of Nursing (2002) *Competencies in Nursing: Nurse Practitioners – an RCN Guide to the Nurse Practitioner Role, Competencies and Programme Accreditation*, London: RCN, July.

Scally, G. and Donaldson, L.J. (1998) 'Clinical governance and the drive for quality improvement in the new NHS in England', *British Medical Journal* 317, 61–65.

Schon, D.A. (1987) *Educating the Reflective Practitioner*, San Francisco: Jossey-Bass.

Schon, D.A. (1991) *The Reflective Practitioner: How Practitioners Think in Action*, Aldershot: Avebury.

Stilwell, B. (2002) Interview conducted with Barbara Stilwell, Scientist, Human Resources for Health, Department of Health Services Delivery, World Health Organization, Geneva, 1 July.

Taylor, B.J. (2001) *Reflective Practice: A Guide for Nurses and Midwives*, Buckingham: Open University Press.

UKCC (1992) *The Scope of Professional Practice*, London: United Kingdom Central Council (available through the Nursing and Midwifery Council, London).

UKCC (1999) *Fitness for Practice*, London: United Kingdom Central Council (available through the Nursing and Midwifery Council, London).

UKCC (2002) *Report of the Higher Level of Practice Pilot and Project: Executive Summary*, London: United Kingdom Central Council (available through the Nursing and Midwifery Council, London).

Weinstein, K. (1999) *Action Learning: A Practical Guide*, 2nd edn, Aldershot: Gower Publishing Ltd.

## Further reading

Manley, K. (2000) 'Organisational culture and consultant nurse outcomes: part 1 organisational culture', *Nursing Standard* 14(36), 34–38.

Manley, K. (2000) 'Organisational culture and consultant nurse outcomes: part 2 nurse outcomes', *Nursing Standard* 14(37), 34–39.

## Chapter 3

# Managing medicines

*Lynda Filer*

In the past, the role of the nurse in relation to managing medicines was defined by the administration of medications from a prescription chart written and signed by a registered medical practitioner. However, with the continuing development of the nursing profession, there have been changes to this practice and there are now a plethora of options in medicine management. The term 'medicines management' has been used here, because it can be defined as 'the entire way that medicines are selected,

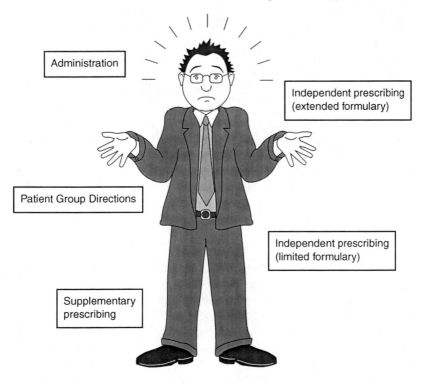

Administration

Independent prescribing (extended formulary)

Patient Group Directions

Independent prescribing (limited formulary)

Supplementary prescribing

*Figure 3.1* The complexity of managing medicines in the nurse-led clinics.

procured, delivered, prescribed, administered and reviewed, to optimise the contribution that medicines make to producing informed and desired outcomes of patient care' (Audit Commission 2001: 5).

The aim of this chapter is to identify the various options available, and to allow the reader the opportunity to reflect upon which may be the most appropriate for his or her own area of practice, and within the nurse-led clinic. The options should not be regarded as a hierarchy, with administration at the bottom and independent prescribing at the top, but have equal weighting depending on the appropriateness to practice and the patient's needs.

## Background

The following section will introduce the various options in managing medicines in chronological order. It will give a brief history of their development, but the detail of each option will be described later in the chapter.

The concept of nurses taking a more active role in the process of prescribing was publicly raised in 1986. *The Cumberlege Report* (DHSS 1986), which focussed on nursing in the community, recommended to the Department of Health and Social Security (DHSS) that nurses should be able to prescribe from a limited list of items. This recommendation was then reviewed by an advisory group that was chaired by Dr June Crown. The first Crown Report was published in 1989 (DOH 1989) and supported nurse prescribing for suitably qualified district nurses and health visitors from a limited list. The Crown Report also recommended the use of group protocols for the supply and administration of medications to patients (DOH 1989). These are now called Patient Group Directions (PGDs) and will be discussed in more detail later in the chapter.

Although it was agreed that some nurses should prescribe, the primary legislation that would allow nurses to do this was passed in 1992, as the *Medicinal Products: Prescription by Nurses Act*. However, the secondary legislation that actually allowed nurses to prescribe came into effect in 1994.

In 1997, it was announced that there would be a review to consider the extension of prescribing to nurses, other than district nurses and health visitors, and to other healthcare professions such as pharmacists. The review team initially reported on the supply and administration of medicines under group protocols, and this report was the first part of Crown II (DOH 1998). In this report, clear criteria were written for establishing group protocols. There was a subsequent change in terminology and the legal term for group protocols became Patient Group Directions (PGDs). The health service circular HSC 2000/026 (DOH 2000) entitled *Patient Group Directions* (England only), enabled PGDs to finally come into practice. Some of the equivalent documents in other parts of the UK were WHC (2000) 116 for Wales (WHC 2000) and NHS HDL (2001) 7 in Scotland (Scottish Executive 2001).

The final report, *Review of Prescribing, Supply and Administration of Medicines* (Crown II), was published in 1999 (DOH 1999). In March 2000, the government announced that it had accepted this report and would take forward the main recommendations, which included extending prescribing powers. Crown II identified two main ways in which this should occur. One was increasing the scope of independent prescribing and the other was 'dependent' prescribing (DOH 1999). This latter term will be discussed shortly.

In October 2000, the Department of Health issued a consultation paper with proposals for the extension of independent nurse prescribing. These proposals included five options for extending the Nurse Prescribers' Formulary. The options ranged from no change in the formulary to all medicines contained in the much broader British National Formulary (BNF). The consultation paper also identified the potential medical conditions where prescribing could be used, and the nurses who may train to prescribe. There were also plans for their preparation and training.

In May 2001, there was a press release announcing the extension of independent nurse prescribing. As in the consultation paper, it identified the medical conditions for which nurses would be able to prescribe treatments. These were minor injuries, minor ailments, health promotion and palliative care. The other key area was identifying what medicines could be prescribed within the remit of those conditions. It was announced that nurses could prescribe, following a period of extended training, all general sales list and pharmacy medicines currently prescribable by general practitioners (GPs), together with a list of around 140 prescription only medicines (POMs). The first nurse training programmes began in January 2002 with the nurses able to prescribe from 1 April 2002.

The second main recommendation from Crown II, as has already been mentioned is that of 'dependent' prescribing (DOH 1999). This term was changed to 'supplementary' prescribing, but the concept remained the same. This indicated that the supplementary prescriber would prescribe for an individual patient whose condition had been diagnosed and a treatment plan drawn up by a doctor, who is the Independent Prescriber. The legislation that allows Ministers to designate new categories of prescribers and conditions under which they can prescribe, is Section 63 of the *Health and Social Care Act 2001*.

In April 2002, the Department of Health and the Medicines Control Agency issued a consultation paper with proposals for the implementation of supplementary prescribing. These proposals included the definition of supplementary prescribing, the criteria including the clinical management plan, the possible range of medical conditions and the formulary required to treat. Another area of focus was the training required by nurses and pharmacists to be supplementary prescribers.

Plans to introduce supplementary prescribing for nurses and pharmacists were announced in November 2002 and changes to National Health Service (NHS) regulations and amendments to the Prescription Only Medicines Order were implemented to allow prescribing from early 2003.

## Prescribing, supply and administration of medicines – the options

As you read through the following information about the various options available, consider the service you are currently providing to your patients.

## Administration of medicines

This can be considered the 'old fashioned' method of managing medicines and involves the administration of a medication against a 'prescription written manually or electronically by a registered medical practitioner or another authorised prescriber' (NMC 2002: 4). The Nursing and Midwifery Council (NMC) have issued a revised version of the United Kingdom Central Council (UKCC) guidelines for the administration of medicines, however the principles remain the same. Whether a nurse prescribes or administers, the nurse is professionally accountable and should 'know the therapeutic uses of the medicine to be administered, its normal dosage, side effects, precautions and contra-indications' (NMC 2002). Therefore whichever option is chosen, it is important that the nurse works within his or her area of expertise.

## Patient Group Directions (PGDs)

Patient Group Directions were formerly called group protocols (DOH 1998). They are 'written instructions for the supply or administration of medicines to groups of patients who may not be individually identified before presentation for treatment' (DOH 2000). The majority of patients should be treated on an individual basis and therefore PGDs should only be used when they offer benefit to a patient without compromising safety. They can be considered most useful where prescribing fits a predictable pattern, such as for immunisations.

The health service circular 2000/026 (DOH 2000) very clearly states the information that a PGD must contain and who may supply or administer through this method.

A multidisciplinary group should create the PGD and it should be signed by a doctor and a pharmacist, who have both been involved in its development. There should be detailed guidance within the PGD and this

---

**Box 3.1   Patient Group Directions (PGDs) (England only: after Health Service Circular 2000/026: DOH (2000))**

A PGD must contain the following:

- the name of the business to which the direction applies;
- the date the direction comes into force and the date it expires;
- a description of the medicine(s) to which the direction applies;
- class of health professional who may supply or administer the medicine;
- signature of a doctor or dentist, as appropriate, and a pharmacist;
- signature by an appropriate health organisation;
- the clinical condition or situation to which the direction applies;
- a description of those patients excluded from treatment under the direction;
- a description of the circumstances in which further advice should be sought from a doctor (or dentist, as appropriate) and arrangements for referral;
- details of appropriate dosage and maximum total dosage, quantity, pharmaceutical form and strength, route and frequency of administration, and minimum or maximum period over which the medicine should be administered;
- relevant warnings, including potential adverse reactions;
- details of any necessary follow-up action and the circumstances;
- a statement of the records to be kept for audit purpose.

---

should ensure that there is consistent clinical practice. There must also be comprehensive arrangements for storage and security of all medicines.

A number of other health professionals as well as nurses, midwives and health visitors are qualified to supply or administer medicines under a PGD, these include pharmacists, physiotherapists and radiographers. However, any of the above may only do so as a named individual. Although the circular states that an individual should be 'trained' to use a PGD, there are no nationally recognised standards for the training and development of staff. However a more recent study has demonstrated that nurses do appear to supply and administer safely using local PGDs (Brooks *et al.* 2003).

## Independent prescribing

In order to be an independent prescriber, the practitioner needs to have the skills to assess and diagnose, for example within his or her area of clinical practice whether as a district nurse prescribing a wound dressing or a family planning trained nurse prescribing the contraceptive pill.

Within this heading of 'independent prescriber' there are two distinct groups who have different annotations on the NMC register. The distinction is concerned with the formulary that the nurse or health visitor can prescribe from. District nurses and health visitors can prescribe from a very limited formulary, whilst nurses completing a longer course can prescribe from the extended formulary.

## Limited Formulary

The Nurse Prescribers' Formulary is a limited list of drugs and appliances (including 12 POMs aimed at meeting the specific needs of patients in the community). Full implementation of nurse prescribing for district nurses and health visitors commenced in England in 1998. The training was an open learning package with three taught days at a higher educational institution and a final written examination. All qualified district nurses and health visitors were encouraged to undertake this training for prescribing.

The training for the Nurse Prescribers' Formulary is now an integrated module within community specialist practitioner training for district nurses and health visitors. At the time of writing there are more than 22,000 district nurse and health visitor prescribers to date in England (DOH 2002a: 1).

## Extended Formulary

Independent nurse prescribers, following training, can prescribe from the Nurse Prescribers' Extended Formulary (NPEF). This includes all medicines in the Nurse Prescribers' Formulary for district nurses and health visitors, plus all general sales list (GSL) and pharmacy (P) medicines currently prescribable at NHS expense. This is in addition to a range of POMs. The medicines can be prescribed in the management of conditions in four specific therapeutic areas:

- minor ailments;
- minor injuries;
- health promotion;
- palliative care.

There is a full list of indications in the extended formulary but they include (see Box 3.2):

---

**Box 3.2 Conditions for which independent prescribers can prescribe from the Nurse Prescribers' Extended Formulary (NPEF)**

*Minor ailments and injuries*
- Circulatory – haemorrhoids
- Digestive – constipation; heartburn; stomatitis
- Eye – conjunctivitis
- Ear – otitis media; wax in ear
- Musculoskeletal – back pain – acute, uncomplicated; soft tissue injury; sprains
- Respiratory – sinusitis; tonsillitis
- Skin – acne; candidiasis
- Urinary System – urinary tract infection (women) – lower, uncomplicated
- Genital Systems – candidiasis – vulvovaginal

*Health promotion*
- Contraception
- Emergency contraception
- Routine childhood and specific vaccinations

*Palliative care*
- Nausea and Vomiting
- Fungating Malodorous tumours

---

An outline curriculum was developed by the Department of Health and the education programme is called 'the preparation of nurses, midwives and health visitors to prescribe from the extended nurse prescribers' formulary'. Since the curriculum was outlined and developed the formulary is now called the Nurse Prescribers' Extended Formulary (NPEF). This was developed in consultation with the now abolished English National Board for Nursing, Midwifery and Health Visiting (the ENB) and representatives from the medical, nursing and pharmacy professions. The outline curriculum was formally agreed and issued to higher education institutions and the National Health Service (NHS) under cover of an education policy letter early in September 2001. As previously highlighted, those first nurses began the training programme in January 2002 and completed in the following April. Amendments to the Prescription Only Medicines Order and Pharmaceutical Regulations allowed them to prescribe from 1 April 2002.

The training programme, as stated in the curriculum document, is 25 study days with 12 days' supervised practice supported by a registered medical practitioner. There are five assessments. These are a review of portfolio or learning log, an objective structured clinical examination

(OSCE), assessment of practice experience, a multiple choice (MCQ)/ short answer question exam, and an exam essay.

The UKCC had agreed standards for the preparation of nurse prescribers to prescribe from the extended formulary and these were published in September 2001. In November 2001, the National Prescribing Centre produced a document 'maintaining competency in prescribing: an outline framework to help nurse prescribers'.

The selection criteria for nurses was also identified and all nurses carrying out prescribing responsibilities from the NPEF will be first level registered nurses or registered midwives. They need to be in a post in which they will have the need and the opportunity to prescribe from the extended formulary. This indicates that it will directly affect patient care. The other selection criteria includes an ability to study at degree level (Level 3), with at least three years' post-registration clinical experience. Another important criteria, which could limit access to the course, is the availability, willingness and ability of a medical prescriber to supervise and support for the 12 days' learning in practice. The medical prescriber needs to be familiar with the programme and in particular his or her role in supporting the students to achieve the learning outcomes. The university running the programme will provide this preparation of the medical prescriber.

## Supplementary prescribing

Supplementary prescribing has been defined as a 'voluntary prescribing partnership between an independent prescriber and a supplementary prescriber, to implement an agreed patient-specific clinical management plan with the patient's agreement' (DOH 2002b).

The independent prescriber identified in relation to supplementary prescribing must be a medical doctor (or dentist) and they will have assessed the patient and made a diagnosis. The supplementary prescriber must be a registered nurse, midwife or pharmacist who will work closely with the independent prescriber. It is important that there is good communication between the two prescribers, as it is a clinical 'partnership'.

There must be a written clinical management plan, which relates to a named patient and to that patient's specific conditions. The clinical management plan should specify the range and circumstances within which the supplementary prescriber can vary dosage, frequency and formulation, and also when to refer. The plan should be evidence based and make reference to guidelines and agreed treatment protocols. Both the independent and supplementary prescriber should agree this. It also needs to be discussed and agreed with the patient.

Unlike extended nurse prescribing, there are no restrictions on the clinical conditions that the supplementary prescriber can treat, and no specific formulary. The key to supplementary prescribing is the clinical management plan, therefore supplementary is most useful in the management of long-term medical conditions and health needs. Supplementary prescribers can prescribe all general sales list and pharmacy medicines and all POMs, with the current exception of controlled drugs, if the medicines are listed in the individual patient's Clinical Management Plan. The issue of controlled drugs, is currently under review and changes may occur.

The training for nurses is based on that for independent nurse prescribing from the extended formulary, which is the aforementioned 25 study days, plus 12 days' supervised practice. There are additional training days specifically related to supplementary prescribing. These days will need to include the Independent Prescriber, so that both members of this new prescribing partnership can develop skills in writing clinical management plans together.

In conclusion, the various options for managing medicines have been discussed. The key points to remember when reflecting on which is the best option for your area of practice and nurse-led clinic, is to ask yourself the following questions:

---

**Box 3.3  Questions relating to the most appropriate choice in managing medicines**

- Is the method you are using at the moment the best and safest for the patient, helping to maximise choice and access?
- Is it the best use of your nursing skills?
- Would your prescribing fit a predictable pattern, therefore could you consider using PGDs?
- Do you work in an area such as minor injuries or family planning? You can consider independent nurse prescribing from the extended formulary.
- Do you work with patients with long standing health needs? Are you a specialist in the management of asthma, diabetes, heart disease etc? Therefore, could you consider supplementary prescribing?
- Does your area of practice involve controlled drugs?

---

The various options in managing medicines have been identified in a way that has allowed the reader the opportunity to reflect upon what option is the most appropriate for his or her area of practice. Of importance is the need to be what may be termed 'politically aware'. This indicates the need to be aware of and indeed anticipate changes in healthcare practice that may require reflection on current personal practice, and discussion with appropriate others. This allows the opportunity to offer both the highest standard and most appropriate form of care provision to the patient or client group.

## References

Audit Commission (2001) *A Spoonful of Sugar*, Wetherby: Audi Commission.

Brooks, N., Durning, F., Bell, I. and Charles, J. (2003) 'The supply of antibiotics by NHS walk-in centre nurses using PGDs', *Nursing Times* 99(4), 36–39.

Department of Health and Social Security (1986) *Neighbourhood Nursing – A Focus for Care (The Cumberlege Report)*, London: HMSO.

Department of Health (1989) *Report of the Advisory Group on Nurse Prescribing (The Crown Report)*, London: DOH.

Department of Health (1998) *Review of Prescribing, Supply and Administration of Medicines, A Report on the Supply and Administration of Medicines Under Group Protocols*, London: DOH.

Department of Health (1999) *Review of Prescribing, Supply and Administration of Medicines. Final Report (Crown II Report)*, London: DOH.

Department of Health (2000) *Health Service Circular 2000/026. Patient Group Directions (England only)*, London: DOH.

Department of Health (2002a) *Extending Independent Nurse Prescribing within the NHS in England. A Guide for Implementation*, London: DOH.

Department of Health (2002b) *Supplementary Prescribing*, London: DOH.

Nursing and Midwifery Council (2002) *Guidelines for the Administration of Medicines*, London: NMC.

Scottish Executive (2001) *NHS HDL (2001) 7. Patient Group Directions*, Edinburgh: Scottish Executive: Health Department.

Welsh Health Circular (2000) *WHC (2000) 116. Patient Group Directions – Review of Prescribing, Supply and Administration of Medicines*, Cardiff: The National Assembly for Wales.

## Further reading

Courtenay, M. and Butler, M. (2002) *Essential Nurse Prescribing*, London: Greenwich Medical Media.

Humphries, J.L. and Green, J. (2002) *Nurse Prescribing*, 2nd edn, Houndmills, Basingstoke: Palgrave.

## Useful websites

The websites for the Department of Health, the Royal College of Nursing and the Nursing and Midwifery Council are useful in keeping up to date with progress in the areas of nurse prescribing and how this affects both the nursing profession and the individual's practice.

Department of Health – www.doh.gov.uk

Royal College of Nursing (RCN) – www.rcn.org.uk

Nursing and Midwifery Council (NMC) – www.nmc-uk.org

## Chapter 4

# Effectiveness and evaluation of the nurse-led clinic

*Emma Pennery*

---

The rise, over recent years, in the numbers and diversity of nurse-led clinics and services makes it imperative that their benefit both to patients and to the delivery and outcomes of care is clearly established (Armstrong *et al.* 2002). This chapter therefore explores the issue of measuring effectiveness in nurse-led clinics, through the exploration of terms such as evaluation, clinical audit and patient satisfaction. The approaches of the quantitative and qualitative paradigms are discussed, together with practical examples to assist the reader in what can sometimes be seen as a minefield. A justifiable concern commonly associated with nurse-led clinics in various practice areas, is the lack of comprehensive evidence that demonstrates if they actually work; that is, do they facilitate meaningful improvement in service delivery and qualitatively enhance patient care?

Evidently, nurses continue to experience difficulties with ensuring that the care they provide is evaluated effectively (McSherry and Haddock 1999; Salvage 1998). Several reasons probably account for why this rigorous evaluation has not always accompanied nurse-led clinics and these are presented below. First and foremost, nurses have not traditionally been skilled in research methodology (conducting or evaluating research) and have been relatively slow as a professional group in embracing the necessity for devising an evidence base of their own. However, since the *Briggs Report* published over 30 years ago (Briggs 1972), which called for nursing to be a research based profession, there have been gradual changes in nurse education and a resultant expansion in the uptake of all aspects of research culture within nursing (Blomfield and Hardy 2000: 114; Cranston 2002). Slowly, the profession is moving from a reliance on tasks and procedures to interventions that are based on rigorous appraisal of evidence (Crinson 1999). However, the continuing reality is that practitioners such as clinical nurse specialists and nurse consultants still struggle to specifically fulfil the research elements of their roles (Armstrong 2002; McCreaddie 2001) and fully utilise research findings to guide their actions (Trinder 2000: 3).

Second, even with this new knowledge, nurses are not always accorded the time or resources to conduct evaluation activity. A study funded by the Department of Health conducted an exploration of new roles in clinical practice with the broad aim of establishing whether there is a relationship between innovative staff roles and individual or organisational effectiveness. Mapping exercises and in-depth case studies specifically on nursing roles found that their effectiveness was not always formally evaluated and was inhibited by a lack of resources (specifically funding, secretarial support, computers and space), volume of work (leading to time constraints) and opposition from key players (Read *et al.* 1999). More recently, another analysis of case studies of post-holders who undertook nurse-led services within innovative roles worryingly found that *none* had carried out definitive evaluation of these roles. Hence, the authors remind us of the necessity to seek methodology that will facilitate objective evaluation and measurement of outcomes (Armstrong *et al.* 2002).

Third, successful evaluation of nurse-led clinics is reliant on the need for more careful attention to be given to the concept of quality of *care* because it is elusive and rarely well conceptualised in the literature (Girouard 1996: 589). It is notoriously difficult to articulate the art of caring, in other words to explicitly (and scientifically) describe and demonstrate how nurses actually make a qualitative difference to care. Nursing work may be undervalued because of the lack of knowledge (specifically among doctors) about the scope and nature of nursing and because of the recognised difficulties of describing the caring aspects of nursing work in ways that will not be dismissed as trivial (Dowling *et al.* 1995). It is essential that nurses in specialist roles who may be conducting nurse-led clinics relate their work to outcomes for patients explicitly, if they are to be valued by their colleagues, employers and the public (Finlay 2000).

Last, and perhaps most controversial, is that the motivations behind the establishment of nurse-led clinics have sometimes been questioned, in terms of them representing legitimate areas for the advancement of nursing, versus nurses being utilised as the cheaper alternative. This in itself may have hindered the progress or, more importantly, the focus of evaluation as stakeholders with competing agendas perceive opposing reasons for promoting and setting up nurse-led clinics in the first instance. Changes in medical manpower and working hours (NHSME 1991) have resulted in the gradual process of nurses adopting more clinical responsibility. Thus the impetus for change has commonly arisen from altered working practices in medicine rather than in nursing per se. Therefore tensions have arisen between those that recognise and welcome opportunities for practice and professional development and those who are concerned about the medicalisation of nursing and therefore the loss of its intrinsic value (Finlay 2000). Arguably, the desire by one professional group to transfer to another's tasks that they find onerous, especially if such a change will prove cost effective and resourceful, may not have patient care and quality assurance at its core. Clearly, nurses must continue to be flexible and responsive to change if we are to retain control of advanced nursing practice roles. This may ensure that they are truly *nurse-led*, rather than arising from pressurised (or bullied), hurried or badly thought out implementation (Marsden 1995).

Nurse-led clinics have undoubtedly become fashionable in recent years, and a potential pitfall of following current trends is the likelihood of jumping on the same bandwagon without thinking carefully about the essential prerequisites. Transparent and explicit demonstration of quality is no longer a luxury, but rather a mandatory aspect of care provided by all healthcare professionals. The quality assurance process is a clinical and managerial framework which necessitates that staff produce a systematic, continuous process of evaluating agreed levels of care and service provision (St Leger *et al.* 1993: 4). In accordance with this, there have been changes in the approach of the National Health Service with regards to implementation of minimum standards of care and assuring an acceptable quality of practice. Service initiatives are monitored and enforced by the Commission for Health Improvement (CHI) which aims to improve the quality of patient care across England and Wales (DOH 2002). Clinical governance remains an umbrella term for everything that helps to maintain and improve high standards of patient care (RCN 2000). It serves as a framework and encompasses various components such as clinical audit, clinical effectiveness and quality assurance. The combined aim of these is to ensure that quality of care is both demonstrable and applicable to all healthcare providers from all disciplines. Together, they represent visible confirmation of a gathering momentum to ensure that care is clinically effective (Rycroft-Malone *et al.* 2002). Maxwell (1984) proposed criteria for indicating the standard of performance (i.e. quality) in a healthcare setting as effectiveness, efficiency, equity, appropriateness, acceptability and accessibility.

## Clinical effectiveness

Clinical effectiveness in turn may be defined as 'the extent to which clinical interventions ... for a particular patient or population do what they are intended to do, that is maintain and improve health, and secure the greatest possible health gain from the available resources' (NHS Executive 1996a: 45). Clinical effectiveness has three distinct parts; obtaining evidence, implementing the evidence, and *evaluating* the impact of the changed practice (Cranston 2002). Thus rigorous measurement of clinical effectiveness generates evidence on which to base practice and is part of the essential evaluation process that demonstrates whether or not changes to practice are appropriate, effective or efficient, and aims to minimise geographical changes in nursing practice (Rycroft-Malone *et al.* 2002; Newbold 1996).

## Evidence-based practice

Inextricably linked with clinical effectiveness is evidence-based practice (EBP). This is defined as an approach to decision-making in which the clinician employs explicit and judicious use of current best available evidence to decide upon the option which best suits the patient (Gray 1997: 41). EBP remains not only a means of empowering professionals, but also a mechanism to deliver the safest and most effective interventions (Blomfield and Hardy 2000: 122; Trinder 2000: 12). The key components of EBP require one to nurture the culture to allow it to flourish, develop the skills, apply these and then evaluate the skills in practice (Cranston 2002). All professionals, therefore, should measure in some way the impact of their knowledge and skills in relation to the needs of those for whom they provide a service (Humphris 1999). Nurses conducting their own clinics are no exception to this. The emergence of government initiatives that emphasise the necessity of measuring effectiveness, for example documents such as *The New NHS: Modern, Dependable* (DOH 1997) and *A First Class Service* (DOH 1998), reiterate that consumers, managers and clinicians need relevant evidence to be both visible and accessible. Without this they cannot be expected to make judgements about the continuing value of nurse-led clinics and specialist nurses as a whole (Humphris 1999).

## What is evaluation?

In broad terms, evaluation is concerned with judging merit (Phillips *et al.* 1994: 1). Girouard (1996: 570), in the context of advanced nursing practice, defines evaluation as 'the systematic application of research procedures to assess the conceptualisation, design, implementation and utility of health care interventions'.

Evaluation in the context of the health service can be defined as the objective critical assessment of the degree to which services fulfil stated goals (St Leger *et al.* 1993: 1). Thus the purpose of most formal evaluation is to produce evidence that will enable the extent to which the intervention (in this case a nurse-led clinic) positively or negatively influences patient care. The main reason for introducing quality assurance into daily nursing activity is to ensure that the nursing profession is continuously evaluating and improving nursing practice (Koch 1992). It would seem imperative that nurse-led clinics provide a quality of care that is at the very least comparable to what already exists. Therefore, by implication, pre-existing outcomes need to be compared to those arising from the initiation of the nurse-led clinic. The key element of any study of effectiveness is the *comparison* between actual practice and some standard, such as an explicitly stated aim of the service or the achievement of a differently organised service of the same intent (St Leger *et al.* 1993: 12). In other words, evaluation of nurse-led clinics requires attention to comparisons, because if the nurse-led service is considered better, this must be qualified in relation to some baseline measure, something which is all too often lacking (Read *et al.* 1999). Comparison in this context may be with the pre-existing service, which offered a different model of care or to a similar service (i.e. the clinic) but offered by a different healthcare professional (often a doctor).

However, if comparing two professional groups (for example in a randomised controlled trial), one must remember that both professionals do not necessarily work under similar circumstances and therefore the same work pressures. It is therefore necessary to determine if differences in patient satisfaction between the two would remain if identical circumstances were in place (e.g. the same rates of booked consultations) (Horrocks *et al.* 2002).

Therefore evaluation of the *process* as well as the outcome of nurse-led clinics is essential to verify and justify their continued development. This is so that attention is given not only to what promotes the best quality of care but also *why* and *how*. Process refers to the actions and behaviours of nursing staff whilst giving care and encompasses the interaction between the patient and the nurse; that is, the process relates to the manner in which care is delivered rather than to what it results in. For example, a study ascertaining the differences between care from nurse practitioners and General Practitioners in primary care clinics revealed the outcome, in terms of resolution of symptoms, was the same. But the process in terms of information provision and duration of consultation differed, with greater preference for nurses in most instances (Kinnersley *et al.* 2000).

*Outcome* relates to what is actually achieved by the care in measurable terms, such as an improvement in health or wellbeing (Koch 1992). Outcomes are quite different from output! The outcome measures chosen need to be specific to the nurse-led clinic under evaluation and the needs of those patients it serves at that time. St Leger *et al.* (1993: 7) remind us of the necessity to make clear the criteria for evaluation and its relevance to the chosen setting. To illustrate this further they cite an example that evaluation of a new cancer therapy would not be sufficient if it only demonstrated disease regression or survival, without attention to quality of life, patient tolerability, absolute cost and cost compared to best available alternatives. Commonly, outcome relates to the recipients of care (the patients), but in the context of extended nurse roles, it may also be prudent to consider the outcomes for the nurses conducting their own clinics.

The likelihood is that the evaluation of the process and outcome of nurse-led clinics cannot exist independently of each other. A key consideration relates to identifying process and outcomes specifically and wholly related to *nursing* care as opposed to medicine for example.

Commonly cited end points such as improved patient care or patient satisfaction are notoriously vague and nebulous and may therefore become
meaningless if they are not accompanied by measurable and specific
objectives. Without these, a link may be made between an intervention
and an outcome inappropriately. For example, if satisfaction is greater
with a nurse-led clinic, this may be due to shorter waiting times or more
time spent in the consultation rather than being attributable just to the
nurse per se. Of greater value is to elicit what it is that the nurse does differently to the existing service and thus what it is specifically about *nursing*
that enhances the care in that setting. Therefore, if patients are more satisfied with nurse-led care, then the precise factors which lead to this should
be elucidated (Horrocks *et al.* 2002). This takes us back to the concept of
not only *what*, but also *how* and *why* nurse-led clinics may facilitate an
improvement in patient care. If one can demonstrate that nursing care
absolutely has beneficial effects on patient outcomes, then it will
strengthen nursing professionalism as a whole, as well as providing sound
verification for the continual emergence of nurse-led clinics in many areas
of practice. However, if the nurse-led clinic results in an identical outcome,
but patients report greater satisfaction with the process that took them
there, then the decision to continue the nurse-led intervention might rest
on cost comparisons alone (see also section on patient satisfaction).

## Quantitative versus qualitative evaluation

Evaluation may be quantitative or qualitative in its approach. There is an
obligation to balance the appraisal of nurse-led clinics using quantitative
statistical indicators (such as post-operative mortality, waiting times,
length of hospital stay and cost effectiveness) versus the qualitative indicators (such as treatment compliance, patient satisfaction and quality of
life) (Day and Klein 2001). Box 4.1 provides a useful checklist to assist
nurses who are involved in the evaluation of nurse-led clinics to consider
both qualitative and quantitative measures. Difficulties may arise from the
fact that quantitative measures are not always sensitive indicators of
*nursing* interventions (Girouard 1996: 570). Nursing issues will often
pertain to the quality of the lived experience of the individuals and the
meaning and values attributed by them (the patient), which is not always
suited to numerical values and statistical analysis (Hewitt-Taylor 2001). In
broad terms therefore, quantitative measures may provide insufficient
information on what nurses actually do, whereas qualitative measures may
be more akin with nursing values, but may not fit so well with the values of
managers, politicians and doctors (Gavin 1997). Thus they are all too often
given insufficient credit by stakeholders, which may hinder such evaluation
from continuing to take place in the future (McCreaddie 2001). Con-
versely, qualitative methods offer ways of capturing and understanding the

> **Box 4.1    Checklist for evaluation of nurse-led clinics (adapted from Girouard 1996: 583)**
>
> - Has the nurse-led clinic improved the care in that setting as measured by changes in the health status of the clients?
> - What impact has the nurse-led clinic had on traditional measures of quality such as morbidity and mortality in that specific care setting?
> - Has the physical, functional and/or psychosocial health status of the clients improved as a result of the nurse-led clinic?
> - Are the consumers satisfied with the care that they receive from the nurse-led clinic, specifically when compared to the alternatives?

element of improvisation of healthcare as well as enabling consideration of equity and humanity (Dingwall *et al.* 1998).

Therefore it is prudent for nurses to recognise the exigency to evaluate a variety of factors about nurse-led clinics. These would include not only improved quality of patient care, but also the impact for the post holder and for the expansion of nursing (such as improved clinical discretion), as well as the organisational benefits for the Trust or environment in which it takes place (see Box 4.2).

Studies appraising nurse-led initiatives, as well as needing to move from being largely descriptive to an explicitly evaluative model, also need to consider longer-term outcomes as well as the immediate ones. This is because it is vital to maintain and develop competence over time; clearly a one-off measurement will not ensure continued development in the future (Lillyman 1998: 125).

## Patient satisfaction and efficiency as outcome measures

The World Health Organization suggests that key components of quality assurance include patient satisfaction with services provided and the use of resources (or efficiency) (WHO 1989). These will now be considered in turn. In studies that have evaluated the impact of a nurse-led clinic on a specific patient population, the most frequent variable measured is patient satisfaction, which refers to the patients' perceptions of how their care was provided (Koch 1992). Broadly, qualitative data pertaining to patient satisfaction is derived from three main sources (Froggatt 2001), experience (observation), enquiry (interviews, surveys, questionnaires) and examination of documentation/material already produced by others (such as records of complaints and compliments received).

Researchers remain divided as to whether this is a crucial and pivotal outcome measure or a largely meaningless and somewhat crude evaluative

---

**Box 4.2  Examples of variables relevant to the evaluation of nurse-led clinics**

*Impact on the patient*
- continuity of care
- improved health outcomes
- satisfaction
- quality of life

*Impact on service delivery/organisation of services*
- differences between health professional groups
- impact on resources
- safety and acceptability
- source of referral to nurse-led clinic
- numbers of patients seen
- impact on waiting times
- length of consultation
- outcome (referral on, discharge etc.) measured against national performance indicators and clinical guidelines if available

*Impact on nursing*
- training needs for the post holder
- documented activity (for example, the numbers of prescriptions, the numbers of referrals to other professionals)
- impact on other role functions
- response from doctors (long standing boundary disputes about roles and responsibilities between doctors and nurses remain hot political issues (Salvage and Smith 2000)

---

mechanism (McGee 1998: 91). Mimnagh (2002) asserts that patient satisfaction is a notoriously unreliable assessment of the standard of care provided, and urges caution about the commonly held fallacy of assuming care is good if patients like it and bad if they do not. Patient satisfaction is gratifying but not necessarily a useful outcome measure of significant health benefit (Nesbitt 2002). This may be so because satisfaction with a service may not indicate the actual quality of what is provided. Clearly quality in the context of healthcare is more than the consequence of consumer satisfaction since the expectations of consumers may be low and their knowledge limited (Redfern and Norman 1990). Patients will inevitably be making comparisons to their previous experiences of care, which may have been particularly poor, such that even a small improvement will be welcomed. Therefore, whilst it remains of certain importance to the patient to be satisfied, this alone may not ensure an impact on patient outcome; that is, satisfaction reflects patient perceptions of their care rather than a guarantee of a definitive improvement in health. There are also real methodological difficulties with capturing patient experiences

and perceptions in a comprehensive way. Low response rates and respon-
der self selection biases cast doubt on the representativeness or otherwise
of the views collected (Day and Klein 2001).

However, Scotland (2002) contends that the debate concerning the relationship between patient satisfaction and standards of care provided, is
perhaps the greatest difference in the paradigm thinking between nursing
and medicine. Increasingly, nursing researchers are convinced that consumer response may be equally as important as the operational performance (Koch 1992), if not more so. Feedback from patients informs us
about what the actual consumers think of nurse-led care. Indeed, recent
documents from the government lend support to the concept of patient-
centred care. The document *Your Guide to the NHS* (DOH 2001) declares
its intended commitment to *user* involvement and to providing a high
quality health service shaped specifically around the needs and preferences of patients. Similarly, the *NHS Cancer Plan* (DOH 2000) stresses
the importance of empowering patients with choice and control in all
aspects of their care. Ensuring the needs of patients are met necessitates
attention to their preferences. Clearly a system which relies on clinical
experts only deciding on what constitutes quality without the patients
themselves entering this negotiation process is on some level flawed (Koch
1992). Thus a counter argument is to accept that the preferences of
patients do have an impact on their outcomes, if only by influencing compliance with care (Sowden *et al.* 1995). Therefore, there seems an obvious
need to take this into consideration when designing evaluative studies of
nurse-led clinics.

## Clinical audit

Undoubtedly an invaluable tool for the evaluation of nurse-led clinics is
audit. Clinical audit seeks to improve the quality and outcome of patient
care through systematic and critical analysis reviewed against explicit criteria. This allows practice to be modified and change implemented where
indicated (NHS Executive 1996b). Clinical audit of nurse-led clinics should
have clearly defined aims, explicit goals and measurable targets for quality
improvement. Audit can consider the effectiveness of the process of care
and/or the acceptability of the specific outcomes of care in relation to the
desired outcomes. For example Jones (1993) evaluated nurse-led minor
injury clinics by conducting an audit of appropriate versus inappropriate
patient use of services and numbers and accuracy of treatment prescriptions issued by the nurses. The former indicates patient acceptability and
patient perception of a nurse-led service. The latter relates to standards of
care and safety issues. Together they consider organisation of care delivery (process) and appropriateness of prescribed care as well as consumer
perceptions (outcome).

Salman *et al.* (1998: 1) propose that audit has a fundamental role to play in gathering data that can be analysed to evaluate clinical practice outcomes and that it is underpinned by a desire to improve practice. In essence, audit enables the assessment of the effects that any changes in care produce, such that the most convincing audits are those that demonstrate progressive improvements in the services or care provided (Smith 1990). A criticism of clinical audit is that it is often fragmented and may lack an overall strategy and mechanisms of feedback (Day and Klein 2001). The key to successful audit of nurse-led clinics lies in learning to regard audit as a process that will continuously aim to improve quality rather than merely being a one-off measurement. Hence mechanisms for audit are commonly referred to as a cycle or a spiral to emphasise the ongoing nature of the process. Both research and audit are important aspects of evaluative strategies, but are clearly not the same thing. Whereas research can be said to 'seek to discover new information', audit 'seeks to improve care' (Williams 1996).

Another aim of the increasing focus on quality is to ensure that 'services are not only more effective but are also more *cost*-effective' (NHS Executive 1996a: 11). In the current climate within the National Health Service, resource management remains an essential priority, because resources are not infinite and expenditure on new initiatives needs to be justified before it will be approved. In other words cost and value are as necessary to emphasise as are effectiveness and quality (Koch 1992). When considering health service delivery, one cannot focus on a comprehensive measurement of outcomes at the expense of an adequate consideration of the associated costs (Kernick 2000). If cost is one of the most significant influences on service provision and thus on professional initiatives, then nurses must be able to address the question of cost-effectiveness, if specialisation is not to be dismissed as expensive, elitist and outdated (Finlay 2000). However, studies suggest that the financial benefits of innovative nursing roles are generally not being measured (Read *et al.* 1999).

Efficiency relates to the relationship between what resources are used to provide the nurse-led service (i.e. the costs) and the outcomes arising from this expenditure (the benefits) for the service. This is crucial because cheaper may not always equate with better (Phillips *et al.* 1994: 82). There are different approaches to the valuing of resources and robust economic analysis is problematical, so nurses evaluating clinics may require assistance from statisticians or health economists if they are to gather meaningful figures. Humphris (1999) reminds us that economic judgements should be concerned with assessment of value, not just costs. However consideration of costs should take more precedence, as it will inevitably be a major influence in the development of future nurse-led initiatives (McCaffrey Boyle 1995). Of course, cost evaluation can never be used in isolation, because quality encompasses not only the numbers of patients seen in a nurse-led clinic but also what is done with them! Cost efficiency may, of course, not be relevant to patients in terms of their ability to recognise its importance, but providers of nurse-led clinics are accountable to more than just their users.

Appropriate comparisons with other forms and providers of care (Humphris 1999) and the assessment of future potential for a particular nurse-led clinic may also be relevant to evaluating efficiency. This helps to see what could be achieved with further changes or greater input of resources. This involves nurses participating in the consideration of what facilitates improved quality versus what are the barriers to success, such as resources, time and role development restrictions. Whilst it may be necessary to ensure that the resource implications of nursing developments are substantiated and in line with service needs, they should probably not be dictated by these alone (Marsden 1995). However, a greater awareness of cost effectiveness among nurses is probably required. The paucity of good evidence regarding the economic impact of substituting nurse practitioners for doctors needs to be addressed in future research, otherwise changes may be introduced that are thought to be efficient when they may not be so (Horrocks *et al.* 2002).

## Some examples: doing it for real

This chapter has emphasised the importance of conducting evaluation of nurse-led initiatives that employ a range of methodologies to measure numerous variables. These range from the perspective of the post holder, the patients and the organisation. Exemplars of this are detailed below to provide the reader with ideas and frameworks upon which to base their own evaluative work. Two clinical areas and a selection of measuring tools are presented which can be modelled to local service needs and delivery as deemed appropriate.

### Example one

Venning *et al.* (2000) report the findings of a randomised controlled trial that aimed to compare cost effectiveness of clinics conducted by general practitioners (GPs) versus nurse practitioners (NPs) in primary care. Interestingly, a broad range of outcome measures were employed in addition to the cost analysis. The randomised controlled trial as a research methodology is widely considered to be the most rigorous. This is partly because patients have a random chance of being recruited to each group under study, irrespective of any preferences of the healthcare professionals involved. It also ensures that patients with various characteristics that could influence the results are distributed more evenly between the groups

(St Leger *et al.* 1993: 96). In accordance with these principles, the randomisation in this study ensured that neither the receptionist (responsible for identifying potential recruits) nor the patient could determine which professional (GP or NP) they saw. The study was conducted across 20 geographically dispersed practices in England and Wales. This helps to counter the accusation lodged at other evaluative studies that findings may fail to reflect generalisable features, focussing instead on those pertinent to just one centre under study.

The data collected by either the GP or NP for each consultation included details of the patient history taken, diagnosis, examination, tests performed, prescriptions and referrals. The duration of each consultation was also recorded and this incorporated interruptions such as the time taken by NPs to get prescriptions signed, so that an accurate portrayal of time taken for each patient was elicited. The patients completed prevalidated and recognised tools to measure health status and satisfaction with the person conducting their consultation. Statistical models were used to analyse the results from all of the aforementioned end points.

The results pertained to a total of 1,316 recruits who were randomised. These numbers enable greater statistical confidence. However, in reality, many evaluative studies on nurse-led clinics, particularly if not randomised or confined to one centre, will achieve much smaller sample sizes. The findings demonstrated that the NPs spent longer in each consultation, but conducted the same numbers of physical examinations and issued fewer prescriptions than the GPs. This is relevant because it suggests the focus (or process) of the consultation may be different when carried out by a nurse. The scales encouragingly revealed that satisfaction was significantly higher among patients seen by an NP. Interestingly, there were no differences in the costs of the care given by the two groups.

Thus this study successfully employs sound methodology to measure a variety of outcome measures including those pertaining to the process of care, the outcome of care from both a health status and patient perception viewpoint and the costs of care with service delivery in mind. Another example of a randomised controlled trial using a similar selection of end points, and conducted on patients with minor illnesses seen by practice nurses or general practitioners, is reported by Shum *et al.* (2000).

### Example two

Hammond *et al.* (1995) report on an evaluation of the effectiveness of nurse-led clinics for patients with breast disease in the hospital outpatient setting. NPs working in breast clinics commonly take histories, examine, request imaging, perform fine needle aspiration cytology and give patients test results. As in the first example, nurse practitioners were compared to doctors (in this case senior house officers) although patients were not randomised to either. Patient satisfaction and anxiety levels were two end-points and were measured using pre-validated scales. Again, the results demonstrated that patient satisfaction was higher and for patients in whom a cancer was suspected, anxiety was reported as less among those seen by a nurse for their consultation compared with a doctor.

To elicit possible reasons for these differences (establishing the *why*), communication styles between the two healthcare professionals was also elicited by tape recording the consultations and applying a pre-validated model for conversation and interaction analysis. Among other things, this explores the focus of the conversation (such as if it is patient-centred or not). Interestingly 'the nurses were found to give more information and more frequently checked the patients' understanding. Some attempt was made to elicit clinical skills by examining the patients' notes and the letters dictated to the GP following the consultation. In both groups no major deviations from the unit's diagnosis and treatment protocols were found.

A final outcome related to the acceptability of the nurse-led clinic by asking patients their preference for seeing a consultant, a house officer or a nurse practitioner for a variety of different clinical problems. Whilst the consultant was favoured for some situations, patients who had previously been exposed to the NP more frequently selected her/him, demonstrating a change in attitude and acceptability once they had experienced nurse-led care.

This study represents another illustration of evaluative work that seeks to measure numerous endpoints which, once again, pertain to both the process and the outcomes of care. Clearly it only relates to one nurse in one clinic and may not, therefore, be generalisable, but is successful for demonstrating the safety, acceptability and improved service to patients of this particular model of care.

Indeed, my own experience of providing nurse-led follow-up after treatment for breast cancer (unpublished thesis in progress) substantiates the above, with greater satisfaction reported in women seen in the nurse-led clinic when compared with traditional medical follow-up. A randomised controlled trial comparing follow-up by the two professional groups has revealed that key advantages of the nurse-led clinic include improved continuity and greater attention paid to emotional needs and answering questions, thus attending to the issues that women perceive hinder rehabilitation and recovery. Although not always easy to articulate why, women noticed a shift of emphasis from the traditional medical model of physical examination of the breast, to a consultation that focussed on the individual patient and the unique impact of breast cancer on their lives. According to the study, areas that specifically benefit from attention in the nurse-led clinic include management of menopausal symptoms, information regarding lifestyle changes and the opportunity to revisit prognosis and individual recovery. Thus the differences nurses make to the consultation is elicited, avoiding the presumption that when nurses take on medical tasks, traditionally performed by doctors, they merely replicate them in an identical way.

## Concluding thoughts

Clearly then, evaluation is paramount to setting up nurse-led clinics. It seems that to secure their continuing evolution, it is essential to achieve recognition of their contribution to nursing practice, to patients and to healthcare delivery generally. Yet extraordinarily this remains an ongoing and so far largely unresolved challenge. Indeed the lack of research on the outcomes of interventions by (advanced) nurse practitioners undermines efforts to substantiate the role (McCaffrey Boyle 1995). Morally and ethically nurse-led clinics must be considered against the need to protect the public and this alone, raises fundamental questions such as, as an intervention: Do they work? Do their benefits outweigh any risks? And finally, are they cost effective (Humphris 1999)?

One ongoing weakness is that success with operationalisation of nurse-led clinics will depend to a large extent on local variables such as the institution and individual nurses (McCreaddie 2001). Nurses may perform differently in clinics and there is a wide variation in areas of practice, tasks undertaken, and preparation and training of individuals prior to commencing their roles. In addition, they use many different outcome measures, reflecting the difficulties in measuring changes in health outcomes after single consultations (Horrocks et al. 2002). Evidence from single cases may add to the picture but far from completes it. Hence there is a need to devise and use better methods for evaluating different forms of care if the results from such evaluations are to provide useful and reliable information (Humphris 1999; Sowden et al. 1995). Until there is identification and understanding of the essential and generalisable features of new working practices (such as nurse-led clinics) as opposed to features specific to the organisation under study, controlled trials will be of limited value (Dowling et al. 1995).

However, if further encouragement is needed, an appraisal of the, albeit sometimes limited, evidence suggests nurse-led clinics can be highly successful in improving patient care (for example Garvican et al. 1998; Mundinger et al. 2000; Sakr et al. 1999; Shum et al. 2000). An extensive review of nurse-led services provided by nurse practitioners in America suggested that they provided improved quality of care when compared directly to physicians. Evaluation in this study included adequacy of physical assessment, resolution of health problems, assessment of patient satisfaction with, for example, information received and rarity of malpractice claims (US Office of Technology 1986).

A more recently published meta-analysis reveals patients are more satisfied if NPs rather than doctors provide care. It seems NPs spend longer with patients, compile more complete records and are associated with offering more detailed and helpful advice to patients (Horrocks *et al.* 2002). In primary care generally, nurses have been demonstrated to provide longer consultations, arrange more investigations and follow-up, provide more information and elicit greater satisfaction than general practitioners. They are not necessarily cheaper but are as safe in managing certain illnesses (Iliffe 2000).

A proposed source of reluctance to the instigation of nurse-led clinics is that patients may have been reluctant to accept consultations from nurses, preferring, perhaps, to see a doctor for safety or efficiency or because they possess greater knowledge. However, Read *et al.* (1999) found patients were universally supportive of nurse-led services, and appeared to have little concern for the professional origin of the practitioner so long as they valued the care that they provided them with.

To reiterate, outcomes may be categorised by quality (improvements in care, patient satisfaction), quantity (numbers of patients seen) and cost (financial implications) (McCaffrey Boyle 1995). Nurses have an obligation collectively and individually to evaluate nursing care. Robust evaluation and evidence of effectiveness provide a basis for the future, but providing effective services in terms of results and costs requires solid evidence which will not emerge overnight (Humphris 1999). St Leger *et al.* (1992: viii) caution that the evaluation of the effectiveness of health services is rewarding but not easy.

By demonstrating and articulating the differences in care that nurses offer and making visible what nurse-led clinics accomplish, we can ensure that practice is refined further. We can also build upon what it is that makes them better and understand how to further shape services for patients. After all, nurses are in a prime position to respond to the patients' agenda and to ensure that the interests and needs of the patient remain paramount. McCaffrey Boyle (1995) wisely advises that evaluation should be an inherent part of setting up nurse-led clinics, rather than an afterthought. In other words, no nurse-led clinic is complete without it.

# References

Armstrong, S., Tolson, D. and West, B. (2002) 'Role development in acute nursing in Scotland', *Nursing Standard* 16(17), 33–38.
Briggs, A. (1972) *Report of the Committee on Nursing*, London: HMSO.
Blomfield, R. and Hardy, S. (2000) 'Evidence-based nursing practice', in Trinder, L. and Reynolds, S. (eds) *Evidence-Based Practice: A Critical Appraisal*, Oxford: Blackwell Science, pp. 111–137.
Cranston, M. (2002) 'Clinical effectiveness and evidence-based practice', *Nursing Standard* 16(24), 39–43.

Crinson, I. (1999) 'Clinical governance: the new NHS, new responsibilities?', *British Journal of Nursing* 8(7), 449–453.

Day, P. and Klein, R. (2001) 'Commission for health improvement invents itself' (editorial), *British Medical Journal* 322, 1502–1503.

Department of Health (1997) *The New NHS: Modern, Dependable*, London: DOH.

Department of Health (1998) *A First Class Service: Quality in the New NHS*, London: HMSO.

Department of Health (2000) *The NHS Cancer Plan*, London: DOH.

Department of Health (2001) *Your Guide to the NHS*, London: DOH.

Department of Health (2002) *About CHI*, London: DOH.

Dingwall, R., Murphy, E., Watson, P., Greatbatch, D. and Parker, S. (1998) 'Catching goldfish: quality in qualitative research', *Journal of Health Services Research and Policy* 3(3), 167–172.

Dowling, S., Barrett, S. and West, R. (1995) 'With nurse practitioners, who needs house officers?', *British Medical Journal* 311, 309–313.

Finlay, T. (2000) 'The scope of professional practice: a literature review to determine the document's impact on nurses' role', *Nursing Times Research* 5(2), 115–125.

Froggatt, K. (2001) 'The analysis of qualitative data: processes and pitfalls', *Palliative Medicine* 15, 433–438.

Garvican, L., Grimsey, E., Littlejohns, P., Lowndes, S. and Sacks, N. (1998) 'Satisfaction with clinical nurse specialists in a breast care clinic: questionnaire survey', *British Medical Journal* 316, 976–977.

Gavin, J. (1997) 'Nursing ideology and the generic carer', *Journal of Advanced Nursing* 26(4), 692–697.

Girouard, S.A. (1996) 'Evaluating advanced nursing practice', in Hamric, A.B., Spross, J.A. and Hanson, C.M. (eds) *Advanced Nursing Practice: An Integrative Approach*, Philadelphia: WB Saunders, pp. 569–600.

Gray, J. (1997) *Evidence-based Healthcare*, Edinburgh: Churchill Livingstone.

Hammond, C., Chase, J. and Hogbin, B. (1995) 'A unique service?', *Nursing Times* 91(30), 28–29.

Hewitt-Taylor, J. (2001) 'Use of constant comparative analysis in qualitative research', *Nursing Standard* 15(42), 39–42.

Horrocks, S., Anderson, E. and Salisbury, C. (2002) 'Systematic review of whether nurse practitioners working in primary care can provide equivalent care to doctors', *British Medical Journal* 324, 819–823.

Humphris, D. (1999) 'A framework to evaluate the role of nurse specialists', *Professional Nurse* 14(6), 377–379.

Iliffe, S. (2000) 'Nursing and the future of primary care', *British Medical Journal* 320, 1020–1021.

Jones, G. (1993) 'Minor injury in the community', *Nursing Standard* 7(22), 35–36.

Kernick, D. (2000) 'Costs are as important as outcomes' (letter), *British Medical Journal* 321, 567.

Kinnersley, P., Anderson, E., Parry, K. *et al.* (2000) 'Randomised controlled trial of nurse practitioner versus general practitioner care for patients requesting "same day" consultations in primary care', *British Medical Journal* 320, 1043–1048.

Koch, T. (1992) 'A review of nursing quality assurance', *Journal of Advanced Nursing* 17, 785–794.

Lillyman, S. (1998) 'Assessing competence', in Castledine, G. and McGee, P. (eds) *Advanced and Specialist Nursing Practice*, Oxford: Blackwell Science, pp. 119–131.

Marsden, J. (1995) 'Setting up nurse practitioner roles: issues in practice', *British Journal of Nursing* 4(16), 948–952.

Maxwell, R. (1984) 'Quality assessment in health care', *British Medical Journal (Clinical Research Edition)* 288, 1470–1472.

McCaffrey Boyle, D. (1995) 'Documentation and outcomes of advanced nursing practice', *Oncology Nursing Forum* 22(8), 11–17.

McCreaddie, M. (2001) 'The role of the clinical nurse specialist', *Nursing Standard* 16(10), 33–38.

McGee, P. (1998) 'Specialist and advanced practice: issues for research', in Castledine, G. and McGee, P. (eds) *Advanced and Specialist Nursing Practice*, Oxford: Blackwell Science, pp. 87–92.

McSherry, R. and Haddock, J. (1999) 'Evidence-based healthcare: its use within clinical governance', *British Journal of Nursing* 8(2), 113–117.

Mimnagh, A.P. (2002) 'Customer satisfaction is all important?' (electronic letter), *British Medical Journal* 324, www.bmj.com/cgi/eletters/324/7341/819.

Mundinger, M., Kane, R., Lenz, E., Totten, A., Tsai, W.-Y. and Cleary, P. (2000) 'Primary care outcomes in patients treated by nurse practitioners or physicians: a randomized trial' *Journal of the American Medical Association* 283, 59–68.

National Health Service Executive (1996a) *Promoting Clinical Effectiveness: A framework for Action in and through the NHS*, London: Department of Health.

National Health Service Executive (1996b) *Clinical Audit in the NHS*, London: DOH.

NHSME (1991) *Junior Doctors: The New Deal*, London: National Health Service Management Executive.

Nesbitt, I.D. (2002) 'Different interpretations' (electronic letter), *British Medical Journal* 324, www.bmj.com/cgi/eletters/324/7341/819.

Newbold, D. (1996) 'An evaluation of the role of the nurse practitioner', *Nursing Times* 29(22), 45–46.

Phillips, C., Palfrey, C. and Thomas, P. (1994) *Evaluating Health and Social Care*, Houndmills, Basingstoke: The Macmillan Press.

Read, S., Lloyd Jones, M., Collins, K. *et al.* (1999) *Exploring New Roles in Practice (ENRIP): Implications of Developments Within the Clinical Team*, School of Health and Related Research (ScHARR), Sheffield: University of Sheffield.

Redfern, S. and Norman, I. (1990) 'Measuring the quality of nursing care: a consideration of different approaches', *Journal of Advanced Nursing* 15, 1260–1271.

Royal College of Nursing (2000) Clinical Governance: how nurses get involved, London: RCN.

Rycroft-Malone, J., Harvey, G., Kitson, A., McCormack, B., Seers, K. and Titchen, A. (2002) 'Getting evidence into practice: ingredients for change', *Nursing Standard* 16(37), 38–43.

Sakr, M., Angus, J., Perrin, J., Nixon, C., Nicholl, J. and Wardrope, J. (1999) 'Care of minor injuries by emergency nurse practitioners or junior doctors: a random-ised controlled trial', *Lancet* 354, 1321–1326.

Salman, A., Kumar, A. and Tomblin, L. (1998) *Auditing of Breast Cancer Care*, Chichester: Aeneas Press.

Salvage, J. (1998) 'Evidence-based practice: a mixture of motives?', *Nursing Times Research* 3, 406–418.

Scotland, J.L. (2002) 'Np's do not want to replace' (electronic letter), *British Medical Journal* 324, www.bmj.com/cgi/eletters/324/7341/819.

Shum, C., Humphreys, A., Wheeler, D., Cochrane, M., Skoda, S. and Clement, S. (2000) 'Nurse management of patients with minor illnesses in general practice: multicentre, randomised controlled trial', *British Medical Journal* 320, 1038–1043.

Smith, T. (1990) 'Medical audit: closing the feedback loop is essential', *British Medical Journal* 300, 65.

Sowden, A.J., Sheldon, T.A. and Alberti, G. (1995) 'Shared care in diabetes' (edi-torial), *British Medical Journal* 310, 142–143.

St Leger, A.S., Schnieden, H. and Walsworth-Bell, J.P. (1993) *Evaluating Health Services' Effectiveness*, Milton Keynes: Open University Press.

Trinder, L. (2000) 'Introduction: the context of evidence-based practice', in Trinder, L. and Reynolds, S. (eds) *Evidence-Based Practice: A Critical Appraisal*, Oxford: Blackwell Science, pp. 1–16.

US Office of Technology (1986) *Assessment: Nurse Practitioners, Physicians' Assis-tants and Certified Nurse Midwives*, Washington, DC: Government Printing Office.

Venning, P., Durie, A., Roland, M., Roberts, C. and Leese, B. (2000) 'Randomised controlled trial comparing cost effectiveness of general practitioners and nurse practitioners in primary care', *British Medical Journal* 320, 1048–1053.

Williams, O. (1996) 'What is clinical audit?', *Annals of the Royal College of Sur-geons of England* 78, 406–411.

World Health Organization (1989) *Quality Assurance in Health Care*, 1(2/3), Geneva: WHO.

## Chapter 5

# Setting up the nurse-led clinic: a framework for practice

*Richard Hatchett*

This chapter examines the variety of issues that can be considered prior to and during the setting up of the nurse-led clinic. These build both on those explored in the previous chapters, which offer a greater analysis, and also prepare for the final case study chapters. These offer an exploration and application of the following issues from practitioners actively involved in setting up nurse-led clinics. In all of the following areas, it is likely that not all can be applied to the same degree. This may be due to simple pragmatics, the skill mix of the team surrounding the clinic, cost and the need for professional development. What is of importance, is the need to reflect on each and consider how the clinic can both address these and move in the direction of application.

## The aim of the clinic

The primary question is what is the aim of the clinic and what objectives do you have? This needs to be specific and will be useful when considering audit and evaluation. It is important to put the patient and service above professional hierarchies and consider how the clinic aims to improve the current healthcare provision in the specified area. This may include greater access to specific services, reduced waiting times, through to the provision of more flexible healthcare in people's lives. The clinic may aim to provide a referral system for other healthcare providers, and/or a walk-in or drop-in service for the public who meet certain criteria. How will the clinic enhance the working of other team members? Will it mean working together is easier, or do you envisage that the service may create initial friction? How can the latter be reduced?

## What are the criteria for access to the clinic?

There is a need to clearly state which patients and users are eligible to use the service and which are not. This is important so that the service offered to those who need it, is as effective and accessible as possible. It also prevents misinterpretation and inappropriate referrals, whether from other healthcare professionals or from the public themselves. The NHS Walk-in Centres are useful examples in this area, where leaflets are produced outlining in list form the services provided and those which are not.

It is possible that a minority of healthcare professionals may abuse the service by continually making inappropriate referrals. This could be for a variety of reasons, and may include a lack of confidence in their own practice in a particular area, with a misguided belief that the clinic will address a much wider array of patient problems. It is this area where good auditing can identify which practitioners, departments or practices are doing this. It can however produce friction if the new nurse-led clinic has not prepared adequate and clear publicity regarding their service. The chest pain clinics highlighted in the *National Service Framework for Coronary Heart Disease* (DOH 2000) are useful in highlighting a service where succinct and clear referral guidelines help prevent a swamping of the service, with those who may not benefit. These clinics, some of which have been nurse-led, are useful in allowing those with new chest pain to access, from primary care, specialist investigations without a prolonged wait. Patients generally should not be accessing the clinic if they are already diagnosed with cardiac chest pain, and should not be revisiting the clinic. It is used as a unidirectional gateway to speedily access further investigation and gain a definitive diagnosis, through the use of specific patient criteria.

Linked to this is the decision regarding who can refer patients to the clinic and who cannot. Here, hierarchical boundaries and traditions may create issues, so there is a need to think carefully how referrals can produce a better service for the patient. In addition is the consideration of whether differing practitioners actually have the skills to appropriately refer, and to have in place an auditing system to monitor inappropriate referrals. The issue of the skills to refer is made difficult with areas such as the nurse practitioner, where there remains only a more recent move towards regulation with regard to preparation or required competencies. Therefore skills to appropriately refer may vary. As the service progresses, the nurse will become aware of those who are referring to the service and their abilities to do this. It is important to base such access on practitioner skills and not purely on who the person is.

## Publicity

In regard to gaining patients and appropriate referrals, there will be a need to both prepare literature and to visit those practitioners key to the success of the service. This will include visiting those who you may need to refer to and those who may refer into the clinic itself. If appropriate, visiting general practitioners, nurses and members of the primary care team at an initial planning stage and valuing their opinions and input is important.

This allows them to see the benefits of the service and how they can fit into it. Visiting as the service is launched is valuable, but it may be difficult to change elements that could have been addressed at the planning stage. Once the clinic is up and running, it may encroach on time, but personal visits to see how the various teams have benefited or value the service is useful. However, it is likely that auditing and evaluation on a less personal level may be necessary, due to work and time constraints.

Despite the created publicity, the nurse may still find a large array of users access the service, with a need to adapt and re-emphasise elements in the literature as the clinic gets underway. Networking cannot be emphasised enough, and there is a need for the nurse to speak at both professional forums and to local interest groups. The former may be general practitioner (GP), practice nurse, or practice manager forums, basically any group that may refer to, or take referrals from the clinic. This is a valuable way of gaining further feedback from actual and potential users, and is a chance to clarify misconceptions and answer questions that may not have been dealt with previously.

## Professional development

Is there a job description created for the nurse(s) running the clinic? Is it possible to break this apart into measurable competencies and to create a realistic education/training plan? Is there a clear knowledge of how to write and use competencies? Are competencies the best approach for practice development? It is of value, as highlighted in this book, to self assess against the created competencies necessary to run the clinic. This will allow the nurse to consider where the priorities for education lie, and also to stage the development of the clinic if an expansion or refinement of the service is envisaged.

Are there strong links with higher education or do these need to be forged? It is of value to talk to those in the university sector to discuss the approaches necessary for professional development. This will be more beneficial once the role and service have been broken apart into smaller elements. Links with other nurses running similar clinics are of value to reduce professional isolation and to help clarify the role.

Are you able to become part of a supervisory relationship? Who might be the best person to approach? It is important to consider the desired outcomes of clinical supervision, because it may not be one person who can provide all of your needs. Do both the participants understand the commitment and role of clinical supervision? Merely meeting for a supportive chat is useful, but the full benefits can only be achieved by planning what will be discussed in the sessions, and making efforts to 'close the gap', that is to take active steps to correct any deficits identified in learning or practice. Can you keep a record of the supervision within your personal portfolio to facilitate professional development? Would group clinical supervision be of benefit to you? Do you fully understand the role and use of reflection?

## Managing medicines

It is important to consider whether the supply or administration of medicines will be a part of the nurse-led clinic. It may not, or it may be that for the service you are providing to be fully effective, you need to reconsider the issue of medicines. Lynda Filer's chapter provides a useful overview of current issues in this area, and asks the reader to consider both their own practice in the clinic and the most appropriate approach to managing medicines.

There is not a hierarchy in this area, with an independent prescriber being regarded as more desirable in terms of skill, than supplying medicines under another healthcare professional's ultimate written direction. It is a case of reviewing the most feasible method of managing medicines for the service the clinic wishes to provide. There is also a need to consider how this will fit in with the role of others managing medicines and associated with the clinic, and the possible evolution of the service. If the current methods are preventing the fulfilment of the clinic's desired care or outcomes, then there is a need to discuss with the manager and other team members, the most appropriate way forward. This will be based on many issues, including the current and future education requirements of the nurse, to the possible need to identify and work with an appropriate team to create a Patient Group Direction (PGD).

## Evaluation and effectiveness

There is a need to consider the issue of evaluating the nurse-led clinic. This can be seen as a minefield, but utilising those within the wider professional community whose roles focus on quality and audit can be invaluable. It is better to utilise a valid tool that has been used before and is therefore reliable, than to reinvent the wheel in isolation. Emma Pennery's chapter explores the various options available, but there is a need to consider both quantifying what the clinic is doing – the numbers seen, time spent with patients, those returning, the specific services offered, and so forth, and importantly evaluation. The latter relates to worth, and there is a need to plan how you can demonstrate that the clinic is effective. This will in part link to the clinic's aim(s) and objectives and may explore patient satisfaction, reduced re-admissions, improved symptom control or increased management of a condition by the patient and/or significant others. It may also be a subsequent reduction in using other health services. Computer programs are increasingly being used to record data as part of an audit and evaluation programme, and accessibility to this form of software can make life a lot easier. There may be a requirement from government or the organisation within which the nurse-led clinic exists to provide statistics, and this needs to be investigated before the clinic is underway. Certainly, documents such as specific National Service Frameworks may have a bearing in this area.

The nurse-led clinic can become restricted by paperwork, and you may need to make a clear case for requiring secretarial support. This is not always available to the clinic, but makes the job both more effective and enjoyable if it can be acquired. It may be necessary to negotiate secretarial support for at least certain aspects of the role or on a part-time basis.

In conclusion and in discussion with those that run nurse-led clinics, it is probably true to say that the nurse needs to be ultra flexible and allow the clinic to evolve. Flexibility may be in the hours worked, through to areas such as professional development, particularly where the clinic evolves to meet the needs of patients who may not originally have been part of the service remit. This is likely in clinics where there are more generalist services, such as the NHS walk-in centres and personal medical services (PMS) sites, but it may affect the more specialist nurse-led clinic too. Such flexibility may mean there is a need to create rapid referral systems, if patients arrive at the clinic with unexpected acute illness. However well planned, it is not until the clinic is running that it can really be seen how it will work and who will wish to use it. The aforementioned issue of networking is useful not only to prevent 'reinventing the wheel' where clinics are meeting the needs of similar client groups, but for colleagues who can offer much needed support when the whole role and service seems overwhelming.

## Reference

Department of Health (2000) *The National Service Framework for Coronary Heart Disease*, London: DOH.

# Case studies

## Chapter 6

# The nurse-led clinic in contraception

*Catriona Sutherland and Shelley Mehigan*

This chapter aims to explore the setting up and running of nurse-led clinics in the field of contraception. The authors have drawn from their extensive experience as expert, specialist nurses and from current and/or core literature. This experience and expertise come from many years of working as clinicians providing contraceptive services in a variety of settings. These include traditional family planning clinics, domiciliary family planning, youth advisory clinics, abortion counselling, community family planning and well woman clinics. In addition, experience has been gained in integrated sexual health clinics and in general practice.

Although it is recognised that men do attend contraception clinics in some settings, they do so in small numbers. The services they access are usually concerned with barrier methods of contraception and sexual problems. They may also support their female partner in her consultation. The authors have chosen to focus solely on the provision of services to and the consultation with the female patient.

The contraception consultation, when it is truly holistic, is highly complex and subtle, having very little clinical skills basis. The consultation is all to do with listening, understanding and asking questions. The skill is in knowing what questions to ask and understanding what the answer might mean.

## The history and development of the nurse-led contraceptive clinic

Marie Stopes (1880–1958) is regarded by many as the pioneer of birth control clinics. Stopes opened the first British clinic in Holloway Road, London in 1921 (McLaren 1992). At this time, only barrier methods were available in the form of caps or diaphragms, condoms and sponges, otherwise there were pessaries, withdrawal (coitus interuptus), douching and the 'safe period'. The safe period is a term that has been used to describe that time in the menstrual cycle when the risk of becoming pregnant is considered low.

Stopes was considerably in advance of her time because she recognised that women would respond more readily to trained nurses than to doctors (Leathard 1980), with any examination and advice being carried out by a qualified midwife. In these early days of birth control clinics, most doctors disapproved very strongly of Stopes' behaviour and beliefs. She defied the medical profession by failing to provide a qualified gynaecologist at all times in her clinic. In addition, not all the birth control organisations were in agreement. Marie Stopes favoured nurses fitting caps and giving advice, while other organisations insisted on doctors doing this. During World War II, in the absence of doctors, nurses found themselves providing services on their own.

By the mid-1970s the Family Planning Association (now the fpa) was the main source of training for doctors and nurses, and the oral contraceptive pill became the most popular method of birth control in England and Wales. By late 1976, in an effort to make the pill more readily available, a Department of Health and Social Security (DHSS) working group recommended that suitably trained nurses, midwives and health visitors, and even some pharmacists, should be able to prescribe the pill (DHSS 1976). This recommendation did not rule out the possibility of pills being available over the counter (OTC) or from slot machines if safer formulations could be developed.

By the late 1970s there were many experienced family planning nurses who were keen to develop their role further. Some enlightened doctors supported advanced training for these nurses. The training given by the doctors was geared to the individual nurses, the needs of the patients and the locality. Some nurses were trained to fit intrauterine devices (IUDs), and also to supply the pill to ongoing users by means of simple protocols. These nurses were working then at a more advanced level than they are now able to do some 25 years later.

What started out as women's clinics or birth control clinics then progressed to family planning clinics. Within the last few years these have developed into contraception and sexual health clinics. Few of those working in these clinics would consider that they are solely concerned with contraception, with most of them now including reproductive and sexual health as part of their remit.

As a result of the evolution of contraceptive clinics, nurse-led services in this field have developed in different ways in different settings. The role of the nurse developed in response to the needs of patients and the demands of the service in that particular setting. Very often the *initial* impetus for the development of a nurse-led service has been the absence of doctors.

Examples of where these clinics have developed include:

- the family planning (FP) trained practice nurse who can provide a holistic service but who needs to have any prescription issued by a general practitioner (GP);
- the nurse working in community based initiatives (domiciliary visiting/community bus/school or college based);
- the nurse working in a designated contraception or family planning clinic;
- the nurse working in a sexual health clinic.

## Nurse-led contraceptive clinics

These aim to:

- improve access to contraceptive care in all settings and to continue providing choice for patients;
- maintain and improve services to those who have particular needs, for example to those who are socially excluded and/or who are very young;
- improve staffing at clinics by making better use of professional skills;
- provide nurses with continuous professional development opportunities developing their skills and expertise.

There are two key aims to the setting up of these clinics:

- to start or to continue to provide a comprehensive contraceptive service, including health promotion, education, sexual health advice and screening;
- to develop and extend the role of the nurse in the contraceptive service in line with the current philosophy of life long learning.

The outcomes should be:

- a comprehensive contraceptive service;
- a holistic service in a safe environment. This complex issue includes: confidentiality and a professional and knowledgeable response to individual needs;
- improved access to services;
- a choice of services for patients.

The nurse who is delivering a nurse-led service should be an experienced contraceptive nurse with recognised competencies. She/he must have been authorised and have been assessed to work to Patient Group Directions (PGDs) within the service, and should undergo regular clinical supervision, appraisal and reflection on their own practice. It is recognised that the term 'regular' can be somewhat nebulous, but a formal structure should be in place to maximise these approaches to professional development. PGDs have been described elsewhere in this text, but were initially recommended

and termed 'group protocols' in the first Crown Report (DOH 1989). They
are specific protocols created by a multidisciplinary team. This includes
medical and pharmacy colleagues, and those professions likely to contribute to care under the protocol. PGDs allow a specific drug to be administered without utilising a practitioner with full prescribing rights, and are
initiated when certain criteria are met (DOH 1998). As part of a subsequent review on the prescribing, supply and administration of medicines,
group protocols were again explored in 1997. This review became the first
part of the second Crown Report (DOH 1999), in which clear criteria were
written for establishing group protocol use (DOH 1998). The health service
circular published in 2000 entitled *Patient Group Directions* (England only)
(DOH 2000), enabled PGDs to finally come into practice.

## Supplying medicines

In considering the more recent past and prior to the Crown committee's
work, protocols, procedures and guidelines entered clinical vocabulary.
Much confusion ensued as their use grew and terminology became
muddled and interchangeable. The increasing use of 'protocols' to enable
nurses to supply medication, without a medical prescription for the specific
individual, raised the issue of whether this practice was in fact legal, and
clarification was sought in relation to the Medicines Act 1968. It soon
became clear that there was no straight answer, because at the time the
Medicines Act came into being no one had envisaged nurses supplying
medicines. Much discussion and debate followed with differing legal opinions on what was actually allowed depending on where, when and who was
supplying or administering which medication.

Most interested parties agreed that it was in the best interests of
patients for nurses to be able to provide supplies of medicines for contraception, but these practices did not fit in strictly with the provisions of the
Act. Different interpretations allowed for doctors to delegate authority to
prescribe/supply/administer in different situations, while definitions of
health service premises became important. Once the issue of legality had
been raised it became more difficult for nurses to continue some otherwise
sensible practices. In an attempt to improve the situation, some senior
nurses and their supporters began developing and using 'group protocols',
applying varying criteria to allow nurses to supply and administer the medications. Unfortunately these varied in quality and effectiveness between
perhaps, one side of A4 paper to a small volume. Many more clinicians
were asking questions, where previously a blind eye had been turned.

The Royal College of Nursing (RCN) and the healthcare union Unison
in particular, lobbied the Department of Health for clarification and eventually the law was amended, with PGDs established as discussed above.
Later still nurse prescribing was extended. The introduction of PGDs

meant that an appropriate system was, and is, now in place for nurses to legally and safely supply and administer medicines. There are still some problems with implementing these as a few doctors and pharmacists (and indeed some nurses) still seem resistant to their introduction despite their governing bodies supporting their use. In addition, some nurses are unable to access and find time and support to undergo training to work with these protocols. Also, despite the law being amended to clarify the legal position, in family planning practice the vast majority of what we do is actually 'supplementary prescribing' (continuing and amending previously prescribed treatment) and does not properly fit into the criteria for PGDs.

Once again we are bending the law to allow us to provide a better service to patients until the further extension of prescribing in all its forms allows many highly qualified nurses to catch up and be able to prescribe within the law. Only when this happens will we truly be able to provide the kind of service to the public that we would like to.

In the field of contraception, PGDs will be produced in line with the needs of the service and the nurses who will deliver that service. This will range from one PGD for emergency contraception (EC) to a variety for supplying pills and administering injections.

PGDs for EC in particular, have been developed in response to a public need for this form of contraception to be made more widely available in non-traditional settings. It has been recognised that nurses who do not have appropriate FP training are capable of supplying EC under a PGD, after having undergone training specific to that group protocol. This has proved to be of great benefit to patients accessing help from nurses in a variety of settings. These include:

- accident and emergency departments;
- NHS walk-in centres;
- schools and colleges;
- genito-urinary medicine clinics.

---

**Box 6.1    Patient group directions in the nurse-led contraception clinic**

Patient group directions are generally used for four purposes:

- to provide a high quality, efficient and acceptable service to patients;
- where the service is to be delivered in a safe environment;
- to improve patient care;
- to maintain and enhance the nurse's professional practice.

In addition, as part of the initiative to improve the access to EC, pharmacists are now able to supply this drug in two ways. Since Levonelle® was granted a pharmacy (P) licence, in addition to Levonelle®-2, the prescription only medicine (POM) version, it is available to all women over 16 at a cost. However, in areas of the country where there is a high teenage pregnancy rate, there are schemes to make Levonelle®-2 available free of charge using PGDs.

Therefore, PGDs for the supply and administration of hormonal contraception (which are available in oral and injectable forms) are needed to enable a nurse-led contraceptive service to function fully. The nurse who is training to work to the PGD should have a recognised qualification and the support of his/her manager.

PGDs for nurses working in contraceptive clinics may include some or all of the following:

- re-issuing of combined oral contraceptive (COC) (this is combined oestrogen and progestogen);
- re-issuing of the progestogen only pill (POP);
- supplying of emergency contraception;
- re-administration of injectable contraception (long-acting contraception);
- initial supply of COC;
- initial supply of POP;
- initial administration of injectable contraception.

There can sometimes be an issue where a patient does not quite fall into the criteria of the PGD to issue the medication. This is where good assessment plays its part, with essentially two broad options. It may be the patient can return another day to see a healthcare professional who can meet their needs. It may be, as in the case of EC, that an answer is needed more imminently. This may be where a telephone link to a medical colleague may be appropriate, but also falls into the remit of knowing when to refer on to a more appropriate person.

Occasionally a patient can backtrack or change the history they have given to more easily fit the PGD. For example, the patient may initially admit to suffering from migraine with aura. They may then change their mind and play down the symptoms in the hope that this may allow them to continue with their method of contraception. It is always important to discuss carefully with the patient the reasons why you are asking the question, and why an accurate clinical history is vital. This emphasises the clinical partnership with the patient you are trying to achieve. It is important to remember that health promotion, in its broadest sense, is an integral part of the contraceptive consultation. Therefore, depending on the education of the nurse and local priorities, there may be PGDs for the treatment and management of some of the more common sexually transmitted infections (STIs), for example, chlamydia.

## Professional development and assessment

Training for nurses in family planning has evolved. Education in this field has always had an emphasis on the clinical component. Originally nurses would sit in with doctors to learn skills and techniques, and with a small number of study days, could gain an FPA certificate. As formal courses developed, more theory was incorporated and these became recognised and validated by a series of institutions and professional groups. These included Introduction to Family Planning, Family Planning Appreciation or Awareness, and advanced family planning courses. These were mostly certificated initially, until the national boards for nursing and midwifery formalised their recognition.

For example the Joint Board of Clinical Nursing Studies course 900 evolved into the English National Board (ENB) 900 and then the ENB 901 and subsequently to the ENB 8103 and their equivalent in other countries. The R71 course was developed when purchasers (most often GPs) in some areas felt that the 8103 did not provide a training that was accessible and appropriate for the needs of their nurses or their clients. It was similar in content and structure to the previous well-regarded 901 and has been run in many areas either instead of or in addition to the 8103. Unfortunately, due to misunderstandings in other areas, it has been wrongly suggested that this did not qualify nurses to work in FP. Additional courses and study days to cater for different groups and to provide training at different levels also developed. The national boards were finally disbanded in 2002.

Two recent developments have combined to change the face of education within this field. One has been the recognition that 'family planning' is an old fashioned term and that sexual activity does not exist in isolation, with a subsequent move towards sexual health and more holistic care. Second, as nurse education has evolved and moved into higher education at advanced level, modular courses are being developed. These have, up until now, tended to include specific national board course elements to allow for recognisable qualifications, which have been what employers and nurses have desired. Now that the national boards have gone and are being replaced by local validated courses within universities, and with moves towards interdisciplinary training within broader areas, this is likely to change even more. For example: women's health degrees and sexual health programmes contain varying amounts of education in issues of infection, contraception, HIV and sexual health promotion, depending on what courses they have evolved from or according to new service demands. It may initially be more difficult for nurses to move from job to job as courses will vary more according to modular content. The learning outcomes may not be so easily transferable and it may be harder for prospective employers to assess the level of skill or competence. This is something we will have to address and is an area where the professional organisations such as the RCN and the Faculty of Family Planning and Reproductive Health Care may need to produce guidance. The guidance would be for minimum competencies and standards in line with those set nationally, such as the Sexual Health Strategy (DOH 2001) and international standards, such as those by the World Health Organization (WHO 2000/2002).

## Managing contraception in practice

It is only by education and continuing professional development that nurses are able to provide the level of knowledge and care that patients deserve. As with all areas of expert practice, the level of skill and knowledge needed to conduct a good contraceptive consultation cannot be underestimated. The knowledge is of the local client groups or groups and their issues. The skill is in asking the correct questions and actively listening to the answers, and to identify what may be termed incorrect answers. These may be identified by what is or is not said, how it is said and by body language. When trying to give unbiased information about methods of contraception and sexual health issues, we should remember that our own verbal and body language may be giving our patients some clues as to our true feelings.

The kind of questions we ask should not give a clue as to the answer we expect, or to the 'right' answer. Using open-ended, rather than leading questions with an implicit answer, is more likely to elicit accurate information and reveal possible problems. Open-ended questions allow the patient the opportunity to participate in and interact in a way that closed questions do not (Parahoo 1997). In the latter, only limited choice is offered, often only requiring a yes or no and doesn't allow the patient to explore or expand on an issue. Box 6.2 offers further suggestions on how to more appropriately phrase questions.

---

**Box 6.2 General advice on more appropriate questioning techniques in the nurse-led clinic for contraception**

| *How not to ask questions* | *How to ask the same questions* |
| --- | --- |
| Are you taking your pills correctly? | Do you remember to take your pills every day? |
| You don't have any problems, do you? | Do you have any problems? |
| Do you start new packs on the same day or is it on different days? | What day of the week do you start new packs on? |
| You do remember to use condoms if you miss a pill, don't you? | What do you do if you forget pills? |
| You don't ever bleed when it's not your period, do you? | Do you bleed other than in the seven-day gap? |

One of the greatest 'miscarriages of practice' in the past has been in the management of women presenting with breakthrough bleeding. Breakthrough bleeding can occur while taking the pill, rather than during the pill-free interval, or at the time of the period (this is relevant when taking the progestogen only pill). This may also be one of the only signs of a STI. Often the response to this was to just change to a different, and sometimes higher dose, pill. This meant that many women who were otherwise happy with their method of contraception ended up being changed from one contraceptive pill to another. Women frequently ended up with the belief that 'the pill does not suit me' or 'I cannot take the pill'. From our experience, many women have obtained their contraception without having much time spent assessing their needs, beliefs, desires and their opinions, and often only being offered the pill, while being unaware of other options. Increased awareness of sexual health and of sexually transmitted infections and the ending of the old fashioned belief that FP patients were what may be termed 'nice women who did not get infections', has led to better treatment and care.

More nurses, particularly those working in general practice, have become skilled in FP and sexual health and this has led to a revolution in care available for women and men. In the past, appointments in general practice for repeat contraception pills were sometimes seen by GPs as 'stop gaps' or 'breathers' in their busy schedule – quick appointments to just check a blood pressure (if the patient was lucky) and no questions asked. Some women have been able to obtain their pills as a repeat prescription over many years, without being seen regularly according to published and generally accepted best practice guidelines. For example: a woman using hormonal contraception should have her blood pressure checked every six months. It is recognised that blood pressure can rise as a result of taking COC and this may be a contraindication. Box 6.3 provides what are termed 'pill rules', issues that should form part of the assessment process for those choosing to use this form of contraception.

---

**Box 6.3   The list of 'pill rules' for use in the nurse-led clinic in contraception**

- When to start the pill
- How to take the pill, including when to stop and restart packets
- When the woman is protected from pregnancy
- When the pill may be less effective
- What to do if a pill is taken late or forgotten
- Issues of concurrent illness
- Possible drug interactions, including over the counter (OTC) products
- What side effects to look out for and why and when to ask for advice

We have found that it is not unusual for women to:

- be taking their pills incorrectly and/or being unaware of the 'pill rules'. As a consequence there is a large group of women who believe they 'became pregnant on the pill'. The 'rules' that women are most commonly ill-informed about are those for missed pills, starting a new pack late, taking other medication(s), diarrhoea and vomiting;
- be suffering from migraine and be taking the pill. This is bad practice because migraine with focal neurological symptoms (formerly known as 'aura') is an absolute contraindication for the combined pill, because it is strongly associated with a risk of stroke. Figures have included an increase in the incidence of ischaemic stroke by about 2.5 times in this group of patients (HEA 2000). Focal neurological signs can be varied, but most commonly present as visual disturbance which resolves prior to the onset of headache. This is generally caused by an interruption in the blood supply to a specific part of the brain;
- have failed to have STIs identified. One study found that chlamydia had been the reason for up to 30 per cent of breakthrough bleeding while on the pill (Krettek *et al.* 1993);
- have not been properly informed of the results of their smear tests;
- wrongly believe that IUDs cause infections;
- have multiple risk factors and 'relative contraindications', which can mean that they should not use their method. This is particularly of relevance in the case of the combined pill and obesity.

Some of these may seem unimportant, but they can permanently affect people's perception of methods of contraception and can mean otherwise perfectly good methods are denied to them because of a mistaken belief that they have failed in the past. Understandably, many women will not use a method that they perceive as having failed.

One of the considerations for nurses, who are not FP trained and who complete the extended prescribing course is that we could end up with a similar situation as in the past, when GPs provided contraceptive services without being appropriately educated. The contraception sessions on prescribing courses may not equate to the level of knowledge acquired by completing a recognised FP course. It is to be expected that nurses' awareness of their accountability will prevent them from prescribing with limited knowledge. However, there are a number of practice nurses currently administering repeat Depo Provera injections (injectable contraceptive) and issuing repeat prescriptions for contraceptive pills to women without PGDs and perhaps not knowing the questions to ask to ascertain whether it is safe to do so. This issue continues to be a real concern. One of the major criticisms of general practice-delivered FP has been the aforementioned lack of education and knowledge of GPs who have always been allowed to prescribe contraception without additional training. If doctors can miss something as significant as a woman suffering from migraine with aura, then so can nurses. It is also important to highlight in this closing section that the nurse should always be aware of the young and vulnerable patient. The nurse would always be considering whether the patient was in an abusive or non-consenting relationship, and would be aware of the local child protection procedures. This is a sensitive area and the RCN have provided useful guidance (RCN 2003). Box 6.4 offers some general considerations in the setting up of the nurse-led clinic in contraception.

## The characteristics of the nurse in the nurse-led clinic

The nurse will have been appropriately educated and will already be working as a specialist nurse. There must also be a willingness to work at this level. The nurse, although working autonomously, cannot work alone all of the time and must also be part of a multidisciplinary team. Peer supervision and opportunities for reflective practice must therefore take place, often informally in the corridor and over lunch, but importantly through a structured approach within formal clinical supervision sessions. This could be with someone chosen from a variety of professions, depending on what the desired outcome of the sessions is to be.

---

**Box 6.4  Setting up a nurse-led clinic in contraception**

Considerations:

- administration – where and when the session will be held, how appointments are to be made, ensuring reception understands the process of access to clinicians and to other services as necessary;
- how the session will be promoted – leaflets, posters, confidentiality statement, any exclusions;
- appointments – by booked appointment or a walk-in service, or a combination, enough time allowed;
- protocols – who can and cannot be seen – sometimes there are upper and lower age limits e.g. under 16s or over 40s, for example pharmacists cannot currently sell EC to those under 16 years of age;
- buying in contraceptives for immediate supply or administration, e.g. Levonelle 2 (EC) or Depo Provera (injectable contraceptive);
- referral systems – for termination of pregnancy (TOP), for specialist contraceptive advice (emergency IUD, contraceptive hormonal implant), treatment and relevant follow up for sexually transmitted infections (STIs);
- measuring the effectiveness of the service. This is an important area and Chapter 4 discusses this issue in more detail.

---

The nurse should have excellent knowledge of local policies, resources, services and agencies. She/he will also have a good knowledge of national issues relevant to the field of practice. It is essential that there is a good network of support set up both within and outside the place of work.

## Sexual history taking

Any nurse in any setting where he/she will be discussing contraception and sexual health, must be able to take a sexual history. Sexual health and contraception are intertwined. Having sex can result in infection as well as pregnancy. A woman needing emergency contraception has, by definition, had unsafe sex and so may be at risk of a sexually transmitted infection.

Sexual history taking is not in itself difficult to learn or do, but is one element of contraceptive and sexual health practice which many people struggle with. This can be for any number of reasons:

- the nurse's own attitude or feelings about questions to do with sex;
- embarrassment for oneself or for the person you are talking to;
- perceived reaction of others to being asked sensitive questions;
- intrusive nature of the questioning into a private area;
- what language to use.

Most people who are experienced in this area will say that they had some or all of these feelings to start with, but do not find it a problem now and that the more you ask the questions and relax yourself, the easier it becomes. Patients can be sensitive to our hesitancy or concern, which they relay back to us. It can be useful to try and practise some questions out loud to yourself, or to a good friend, colleague or partner first and to decide what language you are comfortable using. Essentially this is the valuable use of role play as a method of learning. You will find that when you become used to the language, it will be easier.

All nurses find different things difficult to talk about, but for many nurses the intimate details of sexual activity, sexuality and relationships are the hardest issues to raise and discuss (HEA 2000). It is possible to minimise these difficulties by only asking a question if you know why you need to ask it and what to do with the answer.

## Language tips

Most healthcare practitioners tend to adapt the language they use according to who is sitting in front of them and the same is true in sexual health. There has been discussion as to whether slang or everyday terms are appropriate, particularly with young people and whether one should use these if the patient does, or whether it is better to appear professional and use medical terminology. We generally feel that it is better not to use language you would not normally use yourself, but to use factual and correct terminology. Even young people can find it embarrassing if doctors and nurses start using slang. For example, some people say the more old-fashioned term 'sexual intercourse' or 'intercourse' whereas others prefer just 'sex'. Use of the term 'partner' is usually more appropriate until the nature of the relationship is understood. The information you need helps determine if there are unidentified sexual health issues, fertility control issues or sexual anxieties:

- Is the patient/client having sex? Not everyone is, despite coming to a contraception clinic. If so with whom; bearing in mind this may be more than one person. Do not make assumptions just because you think you know the client. This exercise may be very enlightening for you.
- What gender is the individual or their partner? For example, the incidence of bisexuality is much underestimated and so no assumptions can be made regarding this.
- What sort of sex are they having? Information may be needed concerning safe sex and possible high risk activities.

## What questions/How to ask the questions

How you actually phrase the questions will depend on the situation, how well you know the patient and what he or she has said already. For example, if someone comes asking for emergency contraception you can easily ask: 'When did you have sex?' and then follow this with, 'Who was that with?'

Another useful way of moving onto the subject of sexual activity is to ask about relationships, rather than directly about sex. If you do receive a negative reaction or are asked why you need to know, and in our own experience this very rarely happens and tends to be something nurses expect rather than it being a reality, then you can perhaps ask: 'Are you in a sexual relationship at present?'

---

**Box 6.5 How to make asking difficult questions easier (after the HEA 2000)**

- Only ask questions you need answers to – if you cannot justify a question to yourself, do not ask it.
- Try to normalise the question – say 'I ask everyone this question'.
- Use open-ended questions – let a patient say what they want to say.
- Try to soften what you are saying – say 'Could you tell me...' rather than 'Tell me...'
- Try to elicit the patient's own opinion – say 'What do *you* think the problem is?'
- Use your body language to help a patient feel more relaxed.

- Build up slowly to something that might be really awkward for you or a patient or both.
- Remember the more you ask difficult questions the easier it gets – you learn as you go along.
- It also becomes easier as you get to know a patient – but do not become over familiar.

**Suggested questions to explore risk factors**

How long have you been together?
Do you have sex with anyone apart from your regular partner?
Does your partner have any other sexual partners?
Have these partners been male or female or both?
Have you or your partner(s) spent any time abroad recently?
Do you use protection/condoms?
Do you have oral or anal sex?
Who are you having sex with?
Are you having sex with anyone?
Who is that with?
Where are they from?
Are they from the UK?
Are you still with X?
Have you had sex with anyone else/since your last visit/in the last year?
Who else have you had sex with in the last ... ?
When was the last time you had sex with anyone else?
The latter is quite a useful question, because it could just as easily be 20 years ago as last week.

The above questions are useful in ascertaining a person's risk factors for unplanned pregnancy and STIs. It may also be useful to ask if the patient understands what unprotected sex means? A direct question can be used such as 'What does unprotected sex mean to you?'

## Sexual problems/anxieties

Sex is meant to be enjoyable for both partners, so the contraceptive consultation is an opportunity for disclosure about any kind of problems or difficulties, or lack of knowledge or information. The nurse has a duty to give the patient the freedom to discuss these issues by means of both direct questions and by feedback.

For example:

- Was there anything else you would like to talk to me about?
- You say that you sometimes get a pain with sex: can you tell me more about it?

- You seemed very uncomfortable when I mentioned sex: is there something worrying you?

## Health promotion

Holistic care is fundamental to the contraception consultation and each woman should have her general health assessed. This may include:

- cervical screening;
- breast awareness (issues of breast disorders);
- smoking cessation;
- diet and weight (possible eating disorders, underweight or obese) – a body mass index (BMI) >30 kg/m² is a relative contraindication to the combined oral contraceptive (COC) because of the increased risk of venous thrombosis. Those women weighing more than 70 kg and who take the progestogen only pill (POP) may be advised to double the dose in order to enhance contraceptive effectiveness, even though there is no direct evidence to support this (Camden PCT 2002);
- pregnancy advice, including preconception advice;
- safer sex;
- immunisation;
- STIs;
- significant family history e.g. of thrombosis;
- sexual problems and anxieties.

## Getting prepared

The nurse should only become involved in the nurse-led clinic as part of a willing development. Nurse-led clinics can be seen as expedient in view of doctor shortages in the field of contraception and sexual health. With patient numbers rising, it can be easy to see specialist nurses as a cheap option. The following issues should have been considered prior to starting the clinic:

- the nurse is appropriately educated, has been assessed as competent and is willing to take on the role;
- administration systems are in order;
- supplies and resources are available, for example medications, leaflets, posters, through to larger issues such as the provision of private rooms;
- access to the clinic is established – appointment/walk-in/referral;
- PGDs are prepared;
- inclusion/exclusion criteria of the patients is established;
- referral-onward systems established;

- immediate advice systems established;
- measuring effectiveness/audit set up from the start.

## New drugs

It will be necessary to have set up a system to consider new drugs. These may be defined as those coming onto the market, but also those that are recommended through evidence-based practice for use in specific clinical situations, and may be endorsed by local and national guidelines. This may for example, be through guidelines produced by groups such as the Faculty of Family Planning and Reproductive Health Care or the Royal College of Obstetricians and Gynaecologists. The important issue is to discuss with relevant colleagues, including manager(s) and medical and nursing colleagues the appropriate way forward in managing medicines that best suit the patient's needs. It will also be necessary to consider what further education will be necessary for the nurses who will be supplying or administering the drug(s).

## Running the nurse-led clinic

A key part of the initial consultation will involve general history taking and enabling the patient to choose and use her method of contraception. Remember that hormonal methods of contraception are very safe, as long as those women who have risks associated with these methods have been identified.

Risk assessment is used to identify those at risk of venous thrombosis, arterial thrombosis, or other risks as highlighted above.

Some women will not only be unable to take certain forms of contraception, but may also need to be referred for further investigation/ management depending on what the risk assessment identifies.

For each method of contraception, the nurse will need to know:

- advantages and disadvantages;
- relative and absolute contraindications (WHO (2000) criteria 1, 2, 3 and 4);
- pharmacology;
- mode of action;
- drug interactions;
- likely side effects and their management;
- how to teach the effective use of the chosen method.

There are a few key questions to ask at each pill review:

1   Is the patient still happy with the method?
2   Has the patient stopped the pill or missed taking any?

3　Is the patient taking the pill correctly and consistently?

4　Does the patient understand the risk of extending the pill-free interval?

5　Are there any bleeding irregularities?

6　Does the patient understand that pill withdrawal bleeds are not periods?

In conclusion, this chapter has explored the variety of issues, many still developing, that are relevant to the nurse-led clinic in contraception. A particular emphasis has been placed on protecting the public through sound professional development, but also practice methods such as PGDs that make service provision more flexible to the user's needs. In such a field of work, it is possible to have a close professional relationship with the woman that lasts over many years. The nurse will need to know how to monitor and support ongoing contraceptive use, and be able to care for the woman appropriately as her needs change over time. The expert nurse conducting a contraceptive consultation can make it look deceptively easy. The skill involved should never be underestimated. It is to ensure that the woman is confidently using her chosen method safely and effectively. The nurse is sensitive to all the nuances, both in body language as well as verbally, that might indicate some lack of understanding, incorrect use of method or some possible side effect or other concern, all of which may affect her sexual health and wellbeing. The nurse is in the privileged position of being trusted with the patient's most intimate, personal and sometimes shameful secrets. This is a trust that has to be earned and respected.

## References

Camden Primary Care Trust (PCT) (2002) Standards and Guidelines for the Contraceptive Service, April.

Department of Health and Social Security (1976) *Report of the Joint Working Group on Oral Contraceptives*, London: HMSO.

Department of Health (1989) *Report of the Advisory Group on Nurse Prescribing (The Crown Report)*, London: DOH.

Department of Health (1998) *A Report on the Supply and Administration of Medicines Under Group Protocols*, London: DOH.

Department of Health (1999) *Review of Prescribing, Supply and Administration of Medicines. Final Report (Crown II Report)*, London: DOH.

Department of Health (2000) *Health Service Circular HSC 2000/026. Patient Group Directions (England only)*, London: DOH.

Department of Health (2001) *The National Strategy for Sexual Health and HIV*, London: DOH.

HEA (2000) *Tip cards with supporting effective contraceptive use – a resource for practice nurses*, London: Health Education Authority.

Krettek, J.E., Arkin, S.I., Chaisilwattana, P. and Monif, G.R. (1993) 'Chlamydia trachomatis in patients who used oral contraceptives and had intermenstrual spotting', *Obstetrics and Gynecology* 81 (5 part 1), 728–731.

Leathard, A. (1980) *The Fight for Family Planning*, London: Macmillan.

McLaren, A. (1992) *A History of Contraception: From Antiquity to the Present Day*, Oxford: Blackwell Publishers.

Parahoo, K. (1997) *Nursing Research: Principles, Process and Issues*, Houndmills, Basingstoke: Macmillan Press Ltd.

Royal College of Nursing (2003) *Issues in Nursing: Sign-Posting Guidance Sheet for School Nurses and Other Nurses Working with Young People in Schools and Other Settings About Sex and Relationships*, London: Royal College of Nursing.

WHO (2000) *Improving Access to Quality Care in Family Planning: Medical Eligibility Criteria for Contraceptive Use and Selected Practice Recommendations for Contraceptive Use*, Geneva: World Health Organization.

WHO (2002) *Improving Access to Quality Care in Family Planning: Selected Practice Recommendations for Contraceptive Use*, Geneva: World Health Organization.

## Chapter 7

# The nurse-led clinic for patients following percutaneous transluminal coronary angioplasty

*Alison Pottle*

Coronary heart disease (CHD) remains the major cause of morbidity and mortality in most parts of the industrialised world. Throughout Europe, CHD continues to be the leading cause of mortality in men older than 45 years and in women older than 65 years of age. This remains true despite a decline in the incidence of myocardial infarction (MI) and cardiovascular mortality over the past decades, which is believed to be secondary to the increased recognition of risk factors and heightened public awareness (Tunstall-Pedoe *et al.* 2000). However, as mortality falls, cardiac morbidity is rising due to conditions such as chronic heart failure. The emergence of more effective treatments for acute CHD and the use of prophylactic drug therapies have also had a clinical impact (Sans *et al.* 1997).

Percutaneous transluminal coronary angioplasty (PTCA), with or without the insertion of a stent, has become a widely used and relatively routine practice within cardiology. PTCA involves introducing a balloon catheter, usually via a femoral approach, into a coronary artery which is narrowed by atherosclerosis. The balloon is inflated within the stenosis and assists in widening the lumen to aid blood flow. A stent can be defined as a tiny tubular scaffold placed within a vessel, at a lesion site, to enlarge the lumen and support the vessel wall (Hubner 1998). This may be introduced via the catheter, during the PTCA procedure. The number of PTCAs performed in Europe continues to increase from year to year. The mean European number of PTCAs per $10^6$ inhabitants increased by 22 per cent from 1996 to 1997. In the UK there were 395 PTCAs per $10^6$ population in 1997. This compares to the maximum in Germany of 1,991 per $10^6$ and in contrast, Romania, where the number was 17 per $10^6$ (Maier *et al.* 2002). In addition, in most American and European institutions 60–90 per cent of all PTCA cases now involve stent placement (Stables 1998).

However, the *National Service Framework (NSF) for CHD* (DOH 2000a) identified that the rates of revascularisation, both PTCAs and coronary artery bypass surgery (CABG) in England, were low compared to many other countries. The NSF addressed this challenge by setting a target of increasing the number of revascularisations by 3,000 by April 2002.

Funds were to be invested to enable more effective use of facilities, skills and experience of existing staff. A further increase in capacity would also be needed. The final goal is to have a national figure equivalent to at least 750 PTCAs performed per million of the population. This objective would therefore have implications for service providers in a variety of areas if the complete package of care were to be available to the patients. The NSF also requires hospital trusts to be able to provide 'risk adjusted 30-day and one-year mortality rates for CABG and PTCA'. The need to collect such data is therefore required.

Harefield Hospital is one half of the Royal Brompton and Harefield National Health Service Trust. It is the largest specialist cardio-thoracic centre in the UK and has a national and international reputation for treating patients with heart and lung disease.

At press, approximately 1,000 PTCA were performed in the last financial year at Harefield Hospital. The number has been increasing over the past five years (see Figure 7.1) and this procedure has become one of the main activities within the cardiology directorate. The number is likely to increase further over the coming years.

The post of cardiology nurse consultant was established at Harefield Hospital in June 2000. Nurse consultant posts were born out of three government papers: *Making a Difference* (DOH 1999), *The new NHS Modern, Dependable* (DOH 1997) and *Nurse, Midwife and Health Visitor Consultants* (NHS Executive 1999). Although posts would vary quite considerably between specialities, there are common functions of all nurse consultants (see Box 7.1).

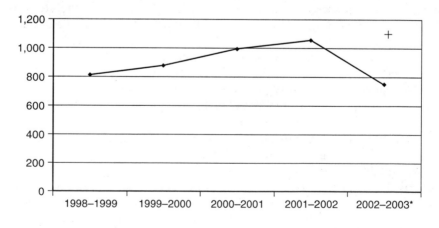

* 2002–2003 April–December only, +=projected number for year end

*Figure 7.1* PTCA numbers: Harefield Hospital 1998–2003.

Core elements of the nurse consultant role:

- help provide better outcomes for patients by improving services and quality;
- provide a career opportunity to help retain expert nurses in clinical practice;
- strengthen leadership in the NHS.

The first Nurse Consultants came into post in April 2000. The cardiology post at Harefield Hospital was the tenth in the country, when I started in June of that year. As this was a new post to me, the hospital and to nursing as a profession, numerous discussions took place as to which areas within cardiology should become part of the role of the Nurse Consultant. The cardiology nursing and medical staff made the decision as to which particular areas should be targeted jointly. Reorganisation of the clinical follow-up for patients after a PTCA was felt to be an important area, which would fulfil a need within the directorate and would also help to launch the new role. Importantly, this new clinic had the potential to meet a perceived care deficit for this group of patients.

The care of patients undergoing PTCA does not just involve the medical procedure, neither does it end when the patient is discharged from hospital. The aim of the clinic is to:

- provide uniform, high quality care to all patients following PTCA;
- fulfil the requirements of the NSF and provide statistics on 30-day and one-year mortality;
- recognise possible restenosis (see below) and facilitate timely reinvestigation;
- provide patients with education, advice and support.

Restenosis or re-narrowing of the coronary artery, which has undergone intervention, is a not infrequent problem and can occur in 32–57 per cent of patients after an initially successful PTCA (Serruys et al. 1994). It is most likely to occur within the first six to 12 months following the

---

**Box 7.1   Nurse consultant functions**

1   Expert practice
2   Professional leadership and consultancy
3   Education, training and development
4   Practice and service development

(NHS Executive 1999)

procedure and is often indicated by a return of the pre-procedural symptoms, most commonly chest pain. It is important that this is recognised early so that investigation, and if necessary further intervention, can be performed as quickly as possible.

This chapter will describe the process of setting up the clinic. Problems, triumphs and initial numbers are included together with plans for further development of the service.

## Development of the clinic

I spent the first six months of my new post carrying out a variety of reviews of current practice within the areas which were to become part of my role, one of which was the PTCA clinic. There are three consultant cardiologists at Harefield and it became evident that no two of them clinically followed their patients in the same way. Following PTCA, clinic visits ranged from being seen once, three months post-procedure and then being discharged, to being followed-up indefinitely. The consultants were also unaware of the practice of their colleagues. I carried out a computer-based literature search through Medline to see if there were any recommendations regarding when patients should be seen in the outpatient department following PTCA, but could find no definitive guidelines. It seemed very much from the literature that the procedure itself carried the most importance and that after care was much less significant.

It was important to have the agreement of all the consultants to the new protocol. This was achieved following a short meeting. Box 7.2 identifies the agreed protocol.

It was generally felt that patients should be seen early after their procedure so that any problems related to the wound site or drug therapy could be addressed. Additionally, seeing the patient early allows for cognitive/behavioural interventions such as lifestyle adjustment and correction of causal misattributions, prior to the behaviour becoming fixed. The six-month appointment would enable patients to be seen at a time when restenosis, if it were going to happen, would frequently have caused symptoms to reappear. The appointment at one year would facilitate the collection of statistics for the NSF as well as monitoring the more long-term outcome for the patients. Continuing to follow the patients for up to five years would enable the collection of a large amount of data on those having undergone PTCA, and would also facilitate the production of local mortality and morbidity figures, a subject which is frequently referred to by the patients.

I decided that the clinics should be run concurrently with the general cardiology clinics. Although the clinic was to be 'nurse-led', I would not be working in total isolation, but as part of the team and I recognised that I would need help and support from the medical staff, especially at the

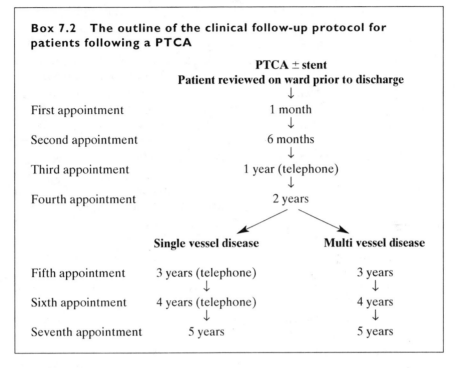

**Box 7.2   The outline of the clinical follow-up protocol for patients following a PTCA**

|  | **PTCA ± stent** |  |
|---|---|---|
|  | **Patient reviewed on ward prior to discharge** |  |
|  | ↓ |  |
| First appointment | 1 month |  |
|  | ↓ |  |
| Second appointment | 6 months |  |
|  | ↓ |  |
| Third appointment | 1 year (telephone) |  |
|  | ↓ |  |
| Fourth appointment | 2 years |  |
|  | **Single vessel disease** | **Multi vessel disease** |
| Fifth appointment | 3 years (telephone) | 3 years |
|  | ↓ | ↓ |
| Sixth appointment | 4 years (telephone) | 4 years |
|  | ↓ | ↓ |
| Seventh appointment | 5 years | 5 years |

beginning. If patients returned to the clinic with chest pain and required further investigation, I needed to have someone I could refer to easily without increasing the time the patient spent in the clinic. A room was available in the outpatient department twice a week, on Tuesday morning and Wednesday afternoon, which coincided with two of the consultant's clinics. The third consultant undertook less intervention than the other two so I felt that, at least initially, his patients could be seen in one of the other clinics. He was in agreement with this. When planning the other aspects of my job, which were more flexible, I had to work around this availability.

It was important that the nurse-led clinic was accepted by all members of staff and afforded a similar status to the medical clinics. I discussed the management of the clinics with the outpatient staff who agreed that the notes would be obtained from the medical records department in the same way as for the medical clinics. An outpatient nurse would be allocated to the clinic to facilitate its smooth running.

Each patient visit would generate a letter for the general practitioner (GP), so I needed to secure some secretarial support. With my other commitments I would not have time to type letters and I felt quite strongly that this was not part of my role. Following a discussion with the business manager, it was agreed that my letters would be typed along with those from the medical staff. This meant that I had to learn the skill of using a dictaphone, which initially I found somewhat strange. However, the secretaries seemed to be able to translate my garble into a meaningful letter. This has resulted in a change of practice for the GPs who are used to receiving clinic letters only from medical staff. Initially there were a few GPs who wrote back to the consultant if they had questions, but now they send most of their letters directly to me. I did not specifically take steps to gain the confidence of these GPs, but time has allowed them to become familiar and used to the change in practice.

Each patient appointment time would be of 15 minutes' duration. In the general clinic patients are allocated 10 minutes, but I felt that the extra five minutes would allow at least some time for discussion of health promotion aspects of care. This is one of the main areas which frequently distinguishes nurse-led clinics from those run by medical staff. Nurses appear generally more holistic in their approach and will ensure that aspects such as personal and psychological issues are addressed.

The format for each appointment was to include a discussion about the patient's general condition, presence of any chest pain or breathlessness, level of activity, employment status, smoking habits, cholesterol level, attendance at cardiac rehabilitation programmes, drug therapy and any concerns the patient may have. Blood pressure would be measured at each visit. The medical consultants agreed the protocol of what would be performed at each clinic visit. Patients would attend the cardiology department prior to the clinic appointment to have an electrocardiogram (ECG) recorded. This could then be reviewed and compared to previous tracings. Although patients attending the clinic have an established diagnosis in that they have had a PTCA and are therefore known to have coronary disease, the nurse is involved in an element of assessment and diagnosis. A handful of patients have been found to be in atrial fibrillation in the clinic. For some this has been a new problem, but this arrhythmia has also been noticed in patients in whom it was overlooked when they were in hospital. I have therefore been able to recognise an important arrhythmia and ensure treatment is initiated. This has hopefully benefited the patients because prompt treatment of such problems should reduce the risk of further morbidity and improve their quality of life.

Secondary prevention is an important aspect of caring for patients with a cardiac condition. I felt it was important that these issues were discussed at each clinic visit. If patients had stopped smoking, I needed to not only acknowledge this achievement, but also ensure that they had not started again by their next clinic visit. All patients should have their cholesterol checked during their admission. If the result was not in the notes I would organise for it to be checked during the first clinic visit. Levels would be rechecked at subsequent visits if this had not been performed by the GP. This would enable monitoring of individual risk factors and ensure my prompt adjustment of drug therapy if necessary. If patients had not seen the cardiac rehabilitation team prior to discharge and had not therefore been offered a place on a one of their programmes, I would offer to arrange this from the clinic. This ensured that the service was available to as many patients as possible.

A copy of the new follow-up protocol was sent to all the local GPs together with the patient's discharge summary, to inform them of the change in practice. I received no comments from the GPs about this change in follow-up. It was agreed with the Consultants that I would be able to independently request tests such as echocardiograms, exercise, respiratory function and blood tests, and also arrange for patients to be readmitted for angiography if necessary. This certainly demonstrates a change in the role of the nurse, as few had been involved in requesting such procedures. Initially I obtained confirmation from one of the medical staff regarding my proposed plan of care for patients, but more recently I have felt confident in my own decisions and have organised for at least 20 patients to have further angiography, many of who have been found to have restenosis. Results from the nurse-led clinic are now being audited to ensure that patients are being reinvestigated appropriately.

Six months was quite a long time to organise the clinics, but I felt that time invested at this stage would lead to fewer changes being needed at a later date. I was lucky in that I had the support of numerous people within the hospital who were keen to help. Several factors contributed to this. Harefield Hospital is a very innovative organisation, which is used to pioneering new ideas. Introducing a new idea is generally greeted with interest and enthusiasm rather than negativity. I had also been working in a senior position at the hospital for 13 years and was therefore well respected and had gained people's confidence. The consultants felt I had the ability to run the clinics and were therefore happy to give their support. I was after all, to be involved in the management of 'their' patients, so it would not have been possible if they did not agree with the idea.

There has been continued discussion as to whether nurse consultants should manage their own caseload (Elcock 1996). I felt that as far as the PTCA patients were concerned, I could not totally manage their care, because if they needed to be readmitted for an angiogram, one of the medical staff would perform this. In some centres nursing staff are undertaking angiography, but at present this is not something being planned at Harefield. Also, I could not perform the PTCA. I therefore felt that in this area of my job it would not be practical for the patients to be seen to be 'my caseload'. The clinics are nurse-led but the patient's care is shared between the consultant cardiologist and myself.

In addition to the clinic, I had identified another aspect of care for patients following PTCA that could be improved. This involved ensuring the patients were fit for discharge and that they understood the procedure they had undergone. Standard practice was that a member of the medical staff saw patients on the evening of their procedure, which was often not the most appropriate time and patients frequently forgot what was said to them. The following morning they would only see patients who had specifically requested to be seen. If the nursing staff felt that the patient had recovered with no problems they were allowed home. This resulted in patients going home without any documentation in the medical notes that they were fit for discharge.

I decided that I would see all the patients who had undergone PTCA on the morning after their procedure. This enabled me to introduce myself to the patients, so they knew who they would see in the outpatient clinic. In this way there is less separation of nurse-led inpatient and outpatient activities. I also explained the procedure, including the possibility of restenosis and reviewed the post-procedural care for the first month. This included medication, driving restrictions, work and general activity. I have produced a post-procedural advice leaflet which includes a diagram of the coronary arteries, on which I indicate which vessels they have had treated. I then document in the medical notes that the discussion has taken place and confirm the patient is fit to go home. If I have any concerns regarding the patient's condition I will order an ECG or blood tests as appropriate and refer back to the medical staff.

The nurse-led PTCA follow-up clinics were started in January 2001. In the first financial year from April 2001–March 2002, 1,029 appointments took place. The numbers continued to increase in 2002 (see Figure 7.2).

Although some of the patients have attended the outpatient department more frequently than prior to the introduction of the new clinic, removing this group from the general cardiology clinics has hopefully resulted in a reduction in the waiting times for appointments for the latter service. It is difficult to demonstrate this because there are always new patients being referred to the cardiologists, and clinics are always full. However the wait for an appointment in the general clinic is between two to six months depending on urgency. If a patient is referred back to the nurse-led clinic by their GP, they can be seen within two weeks. This new system has therefore benefited at least one group of patients.

Each clinic runs for three hours enabling 12 patients to be seen. As the year progressed it became evident that one person could not see all of the patients as per the protocol and provide the quality of care we wanted. Up to 15 patients were being booked into each clinic with the inevitable need to reduce the amount of time spent with each one. As this went against the whole idea of the nurse-led clinic, I approached the clinical director about increasing the number of nurses running the clinics. I was beginning to suffer from the same problem that plagues all people who work alone, what happens when you are not there? As there were no other staff, the

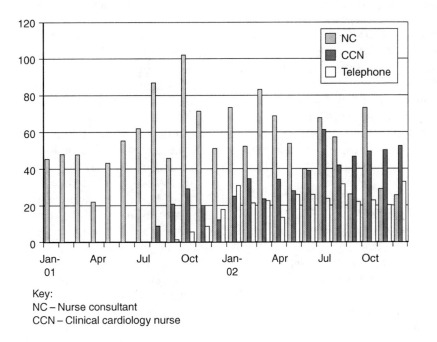

Key:
NC – Nurse consultant
CCN – Clinical cardiology nurse

*Figure 7.2* The number of appointments in the PTCA clinic.

clinics had to be cancelled if I was away. As the numbers increased, patients had their initial appointment at eight weeks rather than one month. This increased the pressure on me and made it virtually impossible to take any holiday. The result was a reduction in my satisfaction with both my job and the way the clinic was running. I began to feel that the clinics had become a production line and a race to see if I could see all the patients in the allocated time.

To ease the strain on the clinics and myself, from August 2001 two additional nurses helped to run the clinics. There was another room available in the outpatient department every Wednesday afternoon and on the second, fourth and fifth Tuesday of each month. The two nurses were experienced cardiology nurses, one working within the research department and one who worked on the ward. They both came to the clinic with me for several weeks to ensure that they were competent and confident about the running of the clinic, prior to them seeing patients on their own. They needed to learn skills in patient assessment and recognition of potential problems following PTCA. Even once they felt confident, I continued to supervise them closely.

At the beginning of 2002 it became evident that there would be a permanent need for additional staff to run the PTCA follow-up clinic.

Coupled with other changes within the cardiology directorate, the clinical director and I decided that we should create a new nursing role. I was asked to write a job description and person specification. This resulted in the role of a clinical cardiology nurse, which incorporates the cardiology research nurse role, but also includes running the PTCA clinics and involvement in non-invasive testing in cardiology. Three posts were created and in July I was able to employ three nurses, two full time and one part time. This has resulted in adequate cover for the clinics for annual leave and sickness and also the introduction of an additional clinic on a Friday morning, which is run by two of these nurses. This clinic runs concurrently with the third cardiologist's general clinic. It is now again possible to see patients at the time intervals stated on the protocol. In addition, the nurses see the patients on the ward before discharge when I am not available. As with the clinics themselves, this aspect of the service was impossible to cover on my own, in addition to my other commitments.

The creation of these new posts has also achieved one of the requirements of the nurse consultant role, which is to develop the service of nursing. However, in creating these posts the question can be raised as to who should be running the clinics? Does it need to be a nurse consultant? If so, we need to change the title of these new nurses. If they, as specialist cardiac nurses can run the clinic, why have a nurse consultant? Much discussion is taking place in nursing regarding titles as alluded to in chapter 1. I feel it is not the title but the nurse and his/her capabilities, which are important in nurse-led services. Experienced cardiac nurses have numerous skills, but running clinics is a different role for most nurses. It is important that they receive adequate training and supervision and that they have a framework in which to work. The nurse consultant role has an emphasis on teaching, particularly for experienced nurses. By educating the clinical cardiology nurses, I was able to not only ensure the patients would receive quality care from suitably trained staff, but also to develop another area of my role.

This expansion of the clinic differentiates it from many other nurse-led services where there is only one nurse running the clinic. This therefore means that services stop if that person is not working. By developing a team we can ensure that the nurse-led clinic is able to run all the time. Nurse-led clinics are still a fairly new idea and not one that was widely used at Harefield Hospital. As such, I feel that it was appropriate for the clinic to be set up by the nurse consultant, as it needed someone with experience and some authority to enable it to happen.

## Telephone follow-up

A relatively new idea for the post PTCA clinic is the concept of substituting telephone follow-up for routine care in the outpatient clinic (Wasson *et al.* 1992). Telephone intervention has been used by other groups to give support and information, but has not been widely used in place of clinic visits (Hartford 2002). It has not previously been used at Harefield Hospital. This novel way of monitoring progress fulfils a variety of needs in the follow-up of PTCA patients. However, there remains a significant risk of restenosis after PTCA, even with the use of some of the newer stents. In view of this, it is important that patients continue to be seen at the interventional centre, so that signs of restenosis can be recognised and acted upon at an early stage.

None the less, all outpatient departments are very busy and it is important not to 'overload' clinics with patients who are perceived to be well to the detriment of those who need to be seen as soon as possible, because of new or continuing symptoms. Patients also frequently have confidence in the centre where their intervention took place. Discharging them from the care of this centre can provoke anxiety and adversely affect recovery. However, it is also important not to promote too much dependence on the hospital.

Telephone follow-up is first performed one year after the intervention. This is arranged as a standard appointment at a date and time convenient to the patient. Patients are generally called at home, but the call can be made to a work or mobile phone number if the patient prefers. Prior to the call, patients are asked to visit their GP surgery to have their blood pressure and cholesterol checked. These results can then be obtained from the patient during the call. The other information discussed is very similar to that addressed during a standard outpatient visit. Calls generally last about 10 minutes. If the patient is showing any signs of restenosis, such as a recurrence of chest pain, an appointment is arranged to see them in the outpatient department as soon as possible. This can usually be arranged within two weeks. If patients continue to progress well, they are followed up as per the protocol. A total of 108 patients have been followed up via the telephone between April 2001 and March 2002.

Patients are not forced to maintain their links with Harefield Hospital. If they prefer to be seen at their local hospital, this can be arranged after the first or second outpatient visit. In practice, most patients have chosen to stay with the Harefield protocol. We aim to follow up all patients over the telephone at one year regardless of whether they have chosen to no longer visit the clinic at Harefield. In developing the telephone follow-up, we have established nurse-led services which are both face-to-face in the clinic, but also at a distance over the telephone. It is possible that this will develop further in the future, employing other aspects of new technology such as video and e-mail.

## Managing medicine

Part of the responsibility in the nurse-led PTCA clinic involves the optimisation of medication. There is evidence from a variety of trials that patients with coronary artery disease have a better outcome if they continue to take medication such as aspirin (Cairns *et al.* 1989) and beta-blockers (Yusuf *et al.* 1988). The National Institute for Clinical Excellence (NICE) has produced clinical guidelines for prophylactic drug therapy for patients following myocardial infarction (NICE 2001). As many of the patients who undergo PTCA have previously suffered an MI, the clinic is a good method of ensuring they are receiving the correct medication.

When I first took up the post of nurse consultant, I discussed with the pharmacists the possibility of producing protocols to enable me to make alterations to medication in the clinic. With the emergence of criteria for establishing group protocols (DOH 1998), and ultimately *Health Service Circular 2000/026* (DOH 2000b), it was necessary for us to modify this to produce Patient Group Directions (PGDs). PGDs allow a specific drug to be administered without utilising a practitioner with full prescribing rights, and are initiated when certain criteria are met (DOH 1998). Their use is further discussed in detail elsewhere in this text.

As with the role of nurse consultant, writing PGDs was new to most of us and therefore took much longer than I had hoped. Luckily, the cardiology pharmacist had some previous experience of writing PGDs in her previous place of work. However, there was no guideline in the Trust regarding whose responsibility it was to write the PGD and I received a variety of conflicting and not particularly helpful pieces of information. In addition, midway through writing the PGDs the Trust decided on a set format, which was totally different to what we had been working on and therefore necessitated even more work.

It took almost two years for the Trust Drugs and Therapeutic Committee to finally approve my PGDs in July 2002. I have since helped to write a document detailing guidelines on how to write a PGD, including what are each individual's responsibilities. Hopefully, this will speed up the process for nurses writing PGDs in the future.

I now have four PGDs, which apply to the various aspects of my role, the content of which was agreed by the cardiologists. Two of these relate to the PTCA clinic. The first enables me to reduce and stop medication in patients who are well following their intervention. When we started writing the PGDs there was much discussion regarding whether one was required to stop medication. I felt quite strongly that stopping drugs was as much 'prescribing' as starting a new drug. This was agreed and the PGD written. Within this direction I am able to stop anti-anginal medication such as nitrates, calcium channel blockers and potassium channel activators if the patient is pain free against the criteria in the PGD. The PGD contains a flow diagram detailing the order in which drugs should be stopped, if more than one is being taken by the patient. I am also able to reduce the dose of beta-blockers, so that patients can be maintained on a dose which affords them the benefit of the drug, with the lowest risk of side effects. This is not strictly part of the PGD, but occurs through a protocol. This is used alongside the PGD.

The alteration of dosages with this PGD also allows for the increase in drugs to ensure therapeutic levels are being taken. This may involve increasing the dose of drugs such as atenolol if the patient is not adequately beta-blocked, or the dose of a statin if the patient has not achieved a satisfactory reduction in lipid levels.

The second PGD enables me to start a limited number of new medications. Included in this are anti-anginal drugs, for patients who are experiencing new symptoms of angina. The PGD also details other actions to be taken in this situation, such as further investigation into the symptoms or readmission for angiography.

Most patients will be discharged from hospital taking aspirin and a beta-blocker, but occasionally this does not happen and the PGD enables me to start both medications. In addition, if patients have a raised cholesterol level, which was not treated whilst they were an inpatient, I can initiate treatment with a statin.

The use of the PGDs is monitored through an audit form. Each time the PGD is used, the relevant form is completed with details of the date, patient details, date of procedure and drugs involved. The pharmacy department will examine these audits annually. The PGDs are valid for two years, at which point they will be re-evaluated to ensure they are still relevant and valid. This will also be a good opportunity to decide if additional drugs need to be added.

There are numerous drugs used within the cardiology setting which could have been included in these initial PGDs. We felt that as this was another new role for both myself and nursing, that it would be prudent to limit the first PGDs to ensure that they worked, before increasing the scope of medications contained within them. It was also difficult to know the extent of drug alteration I would need to be involved in, until the clinics were well established. I was also nervous about extending my role into alteration of medication and was much happier with a more restricted list of medications. The role of nurse prescribing is undergoing further change with the introduction of supplementary prescribing (MCA 2002), which would require further education. This may have an impact on the clinics and will be reviewed as we progress.

After six months of using PGDs, I do feel they have some benefit. They have enabled my patient care to be more holistic. If I feel a patient needs alteration in their medication I am able to do this, without having to wait for a doctor to be available to discuss this with. The result is a more efficient throughput in the nurse-led clinic and also prevents holding up the general clinic. The PGD for altering medication is now to be extended for use by the clinical cardiology nurses. The benefits of nurse prescribing will therefore be extended. This is a natural progression in developing other nurses and expanding their roles. However, it is imperative that all nurses involved in prescribing or utilisation of approaches such as PGDs, have undergone adequate training and assessment, because it is only then that the Trust will indemnify their actions and issues of clinical governance can be adhered to.

I do however have some concerns. The list of drugs within my PGDs is limited. At present there is nothing to distinguish me from a doctor when I complete the drug sheet. Unless the pharmacist is aware of who I am, there is the potential for abuse of the system. There is possibly a need for the status of the prescriber to be stated on the prescription sheet. I could write a drug on a chart, which is not within my PGD and it is possible that the pharmacy would dispense it. This is because I question if all of the pharmacists are aware of what is contained in my PGDs, without referring to them. These are issues which need to be discussed further within the Trust. They also need to be addressed if the use of PGDs is to be expanded.

## Professional development

One of the most difficult aspects of moving into new areas of practice is establishing the levels of competence required. The nurse consultant role is still relatively new and there is no consensus regarding the levels of experience and education required to fulfil such a post. Likewise, the requirements to run a nurse-led clinic are unknown. It is quite difficult to define competencies for roles which are so new and diverse.

I completed an M.Sc. in cardiology a year before I took up this post and feel that I would have been ill equipped to take on this role without the knowledge I gained during the course. Even having studied the subject in some depth, I sometimes doubt my ability to carry out my job. There is always more to learn and I feel I am aware of my limitations and I'm not frightened to ask for help. I am always looking at ways of increasing my knowledge and skills to enable me to give the best possible care to the patients. I work in an organisation which actively promotes continuing education and requests for further study time are viewed positively.

To utilise the PGDs, the cardiology pharmacist and one of the senior registrars assessed my competence. I was asked a variety of questions relating to most of the drugs within my PGDs including indications, contraindications, side effects and interactions. As this was the first time an assessment had been performed, a tool needs to be produced to ensure that the method of confirming competence is valid and reliable.

The *Scope of Professional Practice* (UKCC 1992) has removed some of the barriers which prevented nurses from using their skills. It has enabled nurses to take on roles, which have traditionally been undertaken by doctors, such as running clinics. This has resulted in a blurring of the boundaries between medicine and nursing, but has hopefully achieved the goal of improving patient care.

I am fortunate to have a clinical supervisor who is a senior member of the nursing staff working within the education department of the Trust. For the first few months of my job we met every month, which I found invaluable. Setting up new services is a daunting task and the ability to bounce ideas off someone who did not work within my directorate but who had an understanding of my role and the needs of the service was extremely useful. We now meet every six to eight weeks but often speak in-between times. I also know that if needed, I could request more frequent meetings. I have definitely found clinical supervision useful.

I have also found the exchange of ideas with the clinical cardiology nurses beneficial. Prior to their employment, I was the only one affected by any changes made to the service. They are all keen to take an active role and have had some valuable ideas on how we can take the service forward. I am enjoying being part of a nursing team again, because initially the role of a nurse consultant was rather isolated.

## Measuring effectiveness

There has not yet been a formal audit of the clinics, but comments from patients have suggested that they are satisfied with the service they receive. There remains a lack of understanding amongst the population about what a nurse consultant is, but as many people within the nursing and medical professions find it difficult to explain, this is not unexpected. Patients have however, expressed satisfaction about the fact that the same person sees them each time they come to the clinic. Junior doctors' training dictates that medical staff change their area of work either every six months or every year. Medical clinics are run by a team of staff including senior house officers, registrars and consultants. The consultant is the only permanent member of staff. Therefore the chance of a patient seeing the same member of staff at each appointment is limited. With one nurse, or a small number of nurses running the clinic, there is a much higher probability that this will occur. Indeed, if a particular nurse has seen the patient, every effort is made to ensure that this same practitioner is there for them at their next visit. This therefore enables a much better relationship to be established with the patient and facilitates continuity of care.

Audit of the telephone follow-up is in progress. In the first 12 months of using this method of follow-up, 229 patients have been contacted over the telephone. I have devised an audit tool, which consists of a questionnaire (see Box 7.3), which invites the patients to comment on their views of this method of follow-up and their satisfaction with the service. All the patients have been sent the questionnaire, which has received local ethical approval and has a prepaid envelope to facilitate the form's return once completed. Results from this survey will allow us to measure the effectiveness of telephone follow-up and if the findings are positive, will encourage us to look at further ways of incorporating this method into other clinics in the Trust.

The validity of such audits can be questioned, because the number of replies received limits the results. However, the clinical cardiology nurses are planning to telephone anyone who does not return the questionnaire, so that we obtain as large a response as possible. There will always be the problem that patients may not answer truthfully for fear of a negative response affecting their future care. The letter accompanying the questionnaire explains that this will not happen, but it remains a problem when auditing patient opinions.

---

**Box 7.3    The telephone PTCA follow-up questionnaire**

Are you?                                                                    Male ☐        Female ☐

1    Did you find the telephone follow-up convenient? Yes ☐               No ☐
2    If you had any concerns/problems during the
     telephone call, do you feel they were
     appropriately dealt with by the person you
     spoke to?                                                    Yes ☐               No ☐
3    Was the appointment conducted at the arranged
     date and time?                                              Yes ☐               No ☐
4    Was it easy to remember to be available for the
     telephone call?
              Very easy ☐          Easy ☐         Difficult ☐         I forgot ☐
5    Employment status:
              Working ☐   Retired ☐   Off sick ☐   Unemployed ☐   Medically retired ☐
6    Overall, how satisfied are you with this method
     of follow-up?
              Very satisfied ☐   Satisfied ☐   Neutral ☐   Dissatisfied ☐   Very dissatisfied ☐
7    Would you be happy for some of your
     appointments to be conducted over the
     telephone in the future?                                    Yes ☐               No ☐

Any additional comments:

I have written an additional section to the British Cardiac Interventional Society (BCIS) database, which deals specifically with clinical follow-up. This is a national database set up by the British Cardiac Society to monitor all PTCAs performed in the UK. Patient information is entered onto this following each consultation. Analysis of this data will enable us to assess a variety of aspects of patient care and outcomes following PTCA. As the database was only completed in January 2002, there was a year of data relating to approximately 500 visits, which needed to be entered. The clinical cardiology nurses have been invaluable in doing this and have used the exercise as a way of familiarising themselves with the database. Two years of data is now complete and we are about to start the analysis.

We will now be able to determine our compliance with the NICE guidelines regarding medication (NICE 2001). In addition, it will also be possible to measure the number of patients who attend rehabilitation programmes and to look at the success or otherwise of health promotion, reflected in the number of patients who have maintained desirable cholesterol levels and given up smoking.

Information from the database will enable collection of figures relating to the number of patients who have needed reinvestigation of re-intervention following their original procedure. It will therefore be possible to ascertain the restenosis rate for procedures performed at Harefield Hospital. This information can then be fed back to the Department of Health, but can also be used to inform patients of the likely success rate of the procedure they have undergone.

I feel that the clinic is effective. It has been well received and only three patients have wanted to be seen by a doctor rather than a nurse. Discussions are underway to implement a similar clinic at the Brompton Hospital, the other half of the Trust. Information from the above audits will hopefully provide us with some hard data to support the benefit of the clinic.

## Conclusion and future plans

The purpose of PTCA is two-fold: to improve quantity and health related quality of life. Information from the database will give an indication of the quantity of life post procedure, but there is no measure of quality of life. A research study is to commence next year to look at this aspect of life following PTCA. Research is an integral part of the nurse consultant's role and studies such as this will help expand the knowledge of both medical and nursing staff. Nurse-led clinics offer an exciting opportunity for research studies because they care for a quite specific group of patients.

The number of patients undergoing PTCA is likely to increase in the next few years. It is important that these patients receive adequate follow-up, without duplicating care in primary and secondary care. Many GP surgeries now have nurses employed specifically to perform screening and follow-up for patients with coronary heart disease (CHD nurses). These nurses are well placed to provide the continuing care of patients following PTCA.

A pilot study is planned with a small group of interested local GP surgeries, to set up such follow-up. Patients would have their first two appointments in the outpatient department at Harefield Hospital and would then have their annual follow-up performed over the telephone. Thereafter, the clinical follow-up would be performed at the GP surgery by the CHD nurse. These nurses will be asked to complete a data sheet, which will then be returned to Harefield Hospital for entry onto the database. There will be a section on the bottom of this sheet detailing future follow-up requirements. If the nurse feels that the patient is having symptoms, which warrant review at the hospital, this will be arranged within two weeks. In this way patients will continue to be monitored, but will have a ready access back into the hospital system if problems occur. If this method of follow-up is a success, it will gradually be rolled out to other GP practices.

Nurse-led follow-up for patients who have undergone PTCA has now been in operation at Harefield Hospital for two years. The clinic differs from many nurse-led services which often care for patients with chronic illness, rather than patients during an acute phase of their illness. This system of care appears to have several benefits. It has assisted the cardiology directorate in achieving some of the requirements of audit and reduction in waiting times in outpatient clinics. It appears to have improved patient satisfaction, although formal audit of this has yet to be performed. It has also enabled the development of nurses, specifically the introduction of the role of nurse consultant, but also in the wider expansion of roles within the cardiology directorate. It is also helping to foster new ways of working. Hopefully, this will act as a catalyst for the development of other outpatient services within the Trust.

## References

Cairns, J.A., Singer, J., Gent, M. *et al.* (1989) 'One-year mortality outcomes of all coronary and intensive care unit patients with acute myocardial infarction, unstable angina or other chest pain in Hamilton, Ontario, a city of 375,000 people', *Canadian Journal of Cardiology* 5(5), 239–246.
Department of Health (1997) *The New NHS: Modern, Dependable*, London: DOH.
Department of Health (1998) *The Crown Report 1998. A Report on the Supply and Administration of Medicines Under Group Protocols*, London: DOH.
Department of Health (1999) *Making a Difference: Strengthening the Nursing, Midwifery and Health Visiting Contribution to Health and Healthcare*, London: DOH.

Department of Health (2000a) *The National Service Framework for Coronary Heart Disease*, London: DOH.

Department of Health (2000b) *Health Service Circular 2000/026. Patient Group Directions (England only)*, London: DOH.

Elcock, K. (1996) 'Consultant nurse: an appropriate title for the advanced nurse practitioner?', *British Journal of Nursing* 5, 1376–1381.

Hartford, K., Wong, C. and Zakaria, D. (2002) 'Randomized controlled trial of a telephone intervention by nurses to provide information to patients and their partners after elective coronary artery bypass graft surgery: effects of anxiety', *Heart and Lung* 31, 199–206.

Hubner, P. (1998) *Guide to Coronary Angioplasty and Stenting*, Amsterdam: Harwood Academic Publishers, p. 59.

Maier, W., Camici, P., Windecker, S., Pfiffner, D., Wijns, W. and Meier, B., on behalf of the working group Coronary Circulation of the European Society of Cardiology (2002) 'The European Registry of Cardiac Catheter Interventions 1997', *European Heart Journal* 23(24), 1903–1907.

Medicines Control Agency (2002) *Proposals for Supplementary Prescribing by Nurses and Pharmacists and Proposed Amendments to the Prescription Only Medicines (Human Use) Order 1997*, London: MCA.

National Institute for Clinical Excellence (2001) *Prophylaxis for Patients who have Experienced a Myocardial Infarction – Drug Treatment, Cardiac Rehabilitation and Dietary Manipulation*, London: NICE.

NHS Executive (1999) *HSC 1999/217, Nurse, Midwife and Health Visitor Consultants: Establishing Posts and Making Appointments*, London: NHSE.

Sans, S., Kesteloot, H. and Kromhout, D., on behalf of the Task Force (1997) 'The burden of cardiovascular diseases mortality in Europe. "Task Force of the European Society of Cardiology on Cardiovascular Mortality and Morbidity Statistics in Europe"', *European Heart Journal* 18(8), 1231–1248.

Serruys, P.W., de Jaegere, P., Kiemeneij, F. *et al.* (1994) 'A comparison of balloon-expandable-stent implantation with balloon angioplasty in patients with coronary artery disease. Benestent Study Group', *New England Journal of Medicine* 331(8), 489–495.

Stables, R.H. (1998) 'Routine use of abciximab in coronary stenting?', *Lancet* 352, 81–82.

Tunstall-Pedoe, H., Vanuzzo, D., Hobbs, M. *et al.* (2000) 'Estimation of contribution of changes in coronary care to improving survival, event rates and coronary heart disease mortality across the WHO MONICA Project populations', *Lancet* 355, 688–700.

UKCC (1992) *Scope of Professional Practice*, London: United Kingdom Central Council (available through the Nursing and Midwifery Council, London).

Wasson, J., Gaudette, C., Whaley, F., Sauvigne, A., Baribeau, P. and Welch, H.G. (1992) 'Telephone care as a substitute for routine clinic follow-up', *Journal of the American Medical Association* 267(13), 1788–1793.

Yusuf, S., Wittes, J. and Friedman, L. (1988) 'Overview of results of randomized clinical trials in heart disease II. Unstable angina, heart failure, primary prevention with aspirin, and risk factor modification', *Journal of the American Medical Association* 260(15), 2259–2263.

## Chapter 8

# The nurse-led clinic in diabetes

*Sara Da Costa*

Diabetes mellitus has been recognised as a disease since antiquity (Williams and Pickup 1999: 6). Its definition and the causes of both type 1 and type 2 diabetes are presented in Box 8.1. The discovery of insulin in 1922 was a major breakthrough in the treatment of this disease. Prior to this, patients with diabetes would die a slow and painful death, becoming little more than a living skeleton. They were generally expected to live up to one year from diagnosis (Bliss 2000: 24). Since then, coupled with the development of tablet treatment for type 2 patients, our ability to not only treat diabetes, but also to improve the patients' quality of life has markedly increased.

However, the global incidence of diabetes is increasing in all age

---

**Box 8.1   Definition, types and causes of diabetes**

Diabetes mellitus is a condition in which there is a chronically raised blood glucose concentration.

- It is caused by the absolute or relative lack of the hormone insulin.
- There are two main types of diabetes: type 1, or insulin-dependent diabetes; type 2, or non-insulin-dependent diabetes.
- Type 1 usually presents in childhood and early adult life, and accounts for about 20 per cent of cases in Europe and North America.
- It is thought to be caused by an auto-immune destruction of the insulin producing beta cells in the pancreas.
- Type 2 usually starts in middle age or in the elderly. It is more common, representing about 80 per cent of cases in most European countries and North America.
- It is thought to be due to both impaired insulin secretion and resistance to the action of insulin at its target cells.
- About 80 per cent of type 2 patients are obese.

(Williams and Pickup 1999: 2–3)

groups, including children and young people, and particularly among black and ethnic minority groups, with approximately 1.3 million in the UK currently diagnosed. Many thousands more may have undiagnosed type 2 diabetes, particularly in older people, where the symptoms may be wrongly attributed to ageing (DOH 2001: 6, 9). Diabetes is diagnosed when the fasting blood plasma either exceeds 7.00 mmol/l, or with symptoms and a random blood glucose exceeding 11 mmol/l. Both results require a second raised glucose to confirm diagnosis (Williams and Pickup 1999: 16).

Diabetes is a chronic and progressive disease impacting upon every aspect of life, physically, psychologically and socially. It can result in ill health, disability due to the complications caused by prolonged hyperglycaemia, as detailed in Figure 8.1 and premature death. However, these poor outcomes can be prevented or delayed by high quality care (DOH 2001).

The purpose of this chapter is to explore the role of the Diabetes

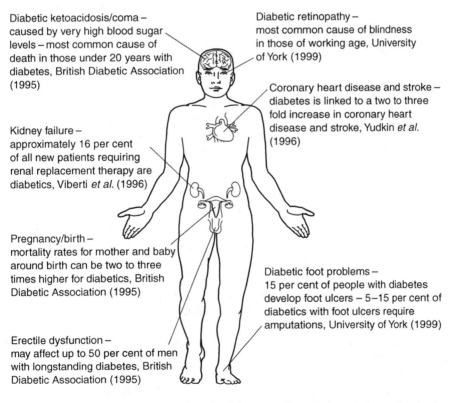

Diabetic ketoacidosis/coma – caused by very high blood sugar levels – most common cause of death in those under 20 years with diabetes, British Diabetic Association (1995)

Diabetic retinopathy – most common cause of blindness in those of working age, University of York (1999)

Coronary heart disease and stroke – diabetes is linked to a two to three fold increase in coronary heart disease and stroke, Yudkin et al. (1996)

Kidney failure – approximately 16 per cent of all new patients requiring renal replacement therapy are diabetics, Viberti et al. (1996)

Pregnancy/birth – mortality rates for mother and baby around birth can be two to three times higher for diabetics, British Diabetic Association (1995)

Diabetic foot problems – 15 per cent of people with diabetes develop foot ulcers – 5–15 per cent of diabetics with foot ulcers require amputations, University of York (1999)

Erectile dysfunction – may affect up to 50 per cent of men with longstanding diabetes, British Diabetic Association (1995)

*Figure 8.1* Complications associated with diabetes mellitus (adapted from the Audit Commission (2000)).

specialist nurse (DSN) in providing this high quality care, in the context of a nurse-led clinic. The majority of these clinics take place in specialist care, that is within acute hospitals, although some do take place within primary care, usually in general practitioner (GP) surgeries. When they do take place in primary care, they are regarded as different to practice nurse-led diabetic clinics because DSNs have a greater knowledge about, and have a singular focus on, diabetes care.

It is important to not only appreciate the breadth and the severity of the problems that diabetes can cause for the individual and their family/loved ones, which will be discussed during these DSN consultations, but also to appreciate that the burden of this disease falls disproportionately on minority ethnic groups and those from socially deprived groups, who have difficulty accessing diabetes services. Therefore, not all patients will have equal access throughout the UK to nurse or medical clinics, although a key element for effective self management is patient education (Audit Commission 2000: 56).

The Audit Commission is an independent body which aims to ensure public money is used efficiently and economically. The Commission's document 'Testing Times' identified a post code lottery for diabetes care (Audit Commission 2000: 107). Post code lottery means that there is a great variation in the way diabetes services are organised and the care that patients receive. This was one of the prompts, along with the rising cost of the condition, to develop a National Service Framework (NSF) for diabetes consisting of specific standards and measurable outcomes. This was in order to raise and make more equitable the quality of care and to improve patient access to services and was subsequently published in 2001 (DOH 2001). An implementation strategy which will identify targets and timescales is in progress. Diabetes care now consumes approximately 5 per cent of total NHS resources and up to 10 per cent of hospital inpatient resources (DOH 2001: 15).

Implicit in the previous paragraph is the notion of variation in terms of standards and needs due to local demographics. This will obviously influence how diabetic nurse-led clinics are provided, but broadly they offer the following opportunities:

- to teach patients about their diabetes, to provide facts in an understandable way and to dispel myths and misconceptions related to their diagnosis;
- to identify achievable strategies for self care, including self monitoring and injecting medication;
- to both empower the patient and follow their agenda;
- to provide surveillance and counselling, enabling lifestyle changes;
- to refer to other members of the diabetes team (primary and specialist care) as required.

This chapter will explore the diabetes nurse-led clinic, drawing from personal experience of a service run in a district general hospital, serving a mainly caucasian population of 300,000 people, which is primarily elderly. The issues discussed throughout this book, including monitoring clinical practice, protecting the public, the legal issues of managing medications and the emergence of the nurse-led clinic will be related to this specific service, within its professional and political context.

## Political context

Most specialist diabetes teams work in diabetes centres within or attached to a hospital. Being part of a hospital means that their set targets must be reflected in our practice. Government initiatives regarding reducing waiting lists and increasing patient access directly affect the care we provide and the processes we use. To encourage these targets being met, Trusts are fined if they fail to achieve, which means there is less money to provide services. This may result in postponements of service development. By meeting the targets, financial penalties can be avoided, which may provide resources instead. There is a considerable evidence base demonstrating that early interventions and aggressive treatment reduce the complications of diabetes (DCCT 1993; UKPDS 33 1998; UKPDS 38 1998). However, despite the publication of the NSF standards (DOH 2001), it is not certain whether additional resources will be available, or whether any related targets may have to be achieved within current budgets.

The difficulty in diabetes, as in many other chronic diseases, is that poly-pharmacy (multiple drugs taken on a daily basis) due to more intensive treatment is becoming more usual, informed by research (UKPDS 33 1998; UKPDS 38 1998) and guidelines from the government body, the National Institute for Clinical Excellence (NICE). This is increasing costs dramatically. Additional staffing will definitely be needed to meet these NSF standards for two main reasons: to educate all involved healthcare professionals to a level that enables best practice, and to cope with the potential doubling of our patient population. This in turn will increase costs but the benefits of these investments will not be seen in the short term, as diabetic complications may take years to develop. Unfortunately, most government policy is designed to demonstrate savings in the short term. What will undoubtedly be needed is collaboration between primary and specialist care to agree care pathways, to agree ownership and to ensure that gaps are identified and filled, and that scant resources are not wasted through duplication.

## Emergence of the diabetic nurse-led clinic

Apart from some innovative posts, the majority of DSN roles were created in the 1980s to provide education for patients on insulin treatment. This was particularly for those who needed to learn how to adjust their dosage as they transferred across to a new insulin strength – 100 units/ml from 20, 40 or 80 units/ml (Da Costa 2000). Once in post and with these transfers completed, DSNs continued to educate patients and healthcare professionals, becoming more involved in direct clinical care within hospital and/or community settings.

Multidisciplinary diabetes teams became more usual in specialist care, while diabetes mini-clinics, often run by practice nurses, emerged in primary care. Payments to practices were made for such chronic disease management clinics. I came into post as a DSN in 1988 and as the only DSN within the health community, began to establish nursing networks of district and practice nurses within the area, setting up courses and becoming a resource for clinical advice. I visited wards to give advice on treatments and provided education for patients and nurses. I also worked for one session with a clinical assistant in the weekly diabetic clinic, providing nursing and educational support. At that time, there appeared to be insufficient demand for a nurse-led clinic.

However, in 1993, a medical consultant diabetologist was appointed and with additional funds for another DSN, a team approach and review of our diabetes service began. We jointly visited GPs and their practice teams to market our specialist care service. This, of course, not only began to increase direct referrals to the consultant diabetologist, but also direct and indirect referrals to the DSNs, because the majority of patients requiring a medical opinion also required some nursing expertise. This involved for example, counselling for lifestyle changes, insulin initiation and adjustment, and blood glucose monitoring. Travel advice, what to do when unwell and adjusting dosage with shift patterns were also common referral requests.

Suddenly, the demand for diabetes nursing increased, and this, along with the need to devise a more time-efficient system than our previous ad hoc appointments, was the driver behind our nurse-led clinics being introduced. Our initial format was four 2.5-hour sessions per week of individualised appointments (two 45-minute, one 30-minute, two 15-minute).

We organised varying appointment lengths in each clinic to meet patients needs. Longer appointments would enable complex problems to be usefully explored, whilst shorter appointments would provide sufficient time for a review of previous advice. Despite waiting lists, our philosophy was and is to provide quality care, which involves useful, uninterrupted time with our patients, identifying their goals and coping strategies. All

DSN clinic appointments were registered on the hospital computer system, which generated appointment letters and illustrated clearly to the organisation one aspect of the nursing contribution to diabetes care.

In comparing these clinics with those which have been set up in part to reduce junior doctors' hours there are interesting differences and similarities. This development happened prior to the emphasis on the reduction in doctors' hours, and was prompted by a need to manage an increasing nursing, not medical, workload. Patients seen in these clinics required nursing skills, not solely a medical assessment, although there is always some overlap in knowledge. Many of the newer specialist posts have been set up purely to take on junior doctors' work, as well as some nursing, and it is hardly surprising that role conflict and confusion is the result (Da Costa 2000).

Many of my DSN colleagues, as well as clinical nurse specialists in cardiology and dermatology, would describe a similar rationale for setting up their nurse-led clinics. Interestingly, the NSF for diabetes (DOH 2001: 5) does not specify the types of clinics and who runs them, other than they should be appropriately trained health professionals. The Audit Commission (2000: 100) stated that those transferring patients to insulin would need specialist support, usually from DSNs, and over time, to identify the right dose and increase patient confidence in self-management. This takes place in our nurse-led group clinic or individual clinic appointment and will be discussed later. Both processes are commonly used by DSNs, dependent on resources (such as physical space and time) and confidence in leading group sessions.

One of the success factors behind the development of our nurse-led clinics has been the support and vision of our medical consultant diabetologist. He has enabled the nursing team to improve patient care by developing insulin dose adjustment protocols through the Trust, by being available to discuss our patients' medical problems and through his confidence in our contribution. Whilst nurses do not always need a medical champion, it can help in developing a more autonomous nursing role. When one profession appears to be advancing more quickly than others in a team, it can begin to blur the boundaries and certainly this is true of doctors and nurses. I would agree with GP Patrick White (2000) who argues that nurses should perform the tasks which they can do better than the doctor, while sharing those that each does equally well. This is rather than the nurse doing those tasks, which he as a doctor dislikes doing, more cheaply and efficiently. Such issues may be the legacy of the reduction of junior doctors' hours.

Part of our development as a nursing team is because we have never been seen as, or see ourselves as, doctors' substitutes. This would have undermined the whole notion of team working, which is surely not about everyone trying to do the same job, but instead celebrating our differences and ensuring patients benefit by seeing the appropriate health-care professional.

The British Medical Association has suggested a new model for NHS care (BMA 2002) emphasising how nurses' skills should be used to their full potential by coordinating the care around a patient, while doctors would concentrate on the areas where their skills can be best used. Nurses view patients holistically, which involves life outside of a hospital or GP practice, which is crucial for appropriate discharge and referral decisions. Doctors would no longer be seen as the lone 'gatekeepers' to care provided by the NHS. In secondary care, the BMA suggests that a clinical nurse specialist would coordinate the care given by other professionals, including doctors and would also have an advanced nursing role. One could argue that some of this is happening already with experienced DSNs and in particular, nurse consultants in diabetes. For example, on the wards, in general practice and in our nurse-led clinics, we advise our medical colleagues (GPs and hospital teams) regarding therapies and review criteria. We also manage our own caseload which includes referring our patients to other specialist areas and teams. This is in line with the chief nursing officer's 10 key roles for nurses, as outlined in Chapter One.

## Managing medications

Patients attending our nurse-led clinics commonly require a review of medications in terms of dose adjustments or additional therapy. DSNs adjust insulin via an agreed hospital protocol, which identifies the insulins used and also the range of dose which can be altered. This is not the same as a Patient Group Direction (PGD), discussed elsewhere in this text, purely because our team's development preceded this and fulfils a need for nurses to advise patients in self-management of their medications. Such therapy issues are discussed between team members as they occur, and if a trend emerges, may be discussed in more detail at our weekly team meetings.

Patients taking oral hypoglycaemic tablets can have their doses altered within and up to their maximum dose at our discretion. We recommend these changes verbally to our patients and then formally in a letter to their GP, or if referred from a hospital team, also to the medical consultant involved. We do not dispense medications from our clinic, instead, all new medication must be prescribed by a doctor in our team and then dispensed at our hospital pharmacy. We do not alter dosages of any drugs other than those specified on our protocol, although that is likely to change given the intensification of drug treatment for our patients and developments in nurse prescribing.

Although medication adjustment by nursing staff without prescribing rights is essentially illegal, the use of hospital protocols, written by a consultant diabetologist, appears to be custom and practice within the UK. Nurse prescribing may increasingly impact on the DSN team through the use of PGDs. This will essentially allow DSNs to administer a certain medication by the use of a protocol, when specific criteria are met, much as we are doing now. Our patients always attend our clinics once diagnosed, so I believe it unlikely that we will need to be independent prescribers. Supplementary prescribing may be helpful to our patients. This, for example, may be through prescribing changes or additions to drugs on the wards. The ramifications of supplementary prescribing have been discussed in Lynda Filer's chapter, so I will not repeat them here, suffice to say that considerations regarding patient benefits, staff resources, and training and support within the team will need to be further explored.

## Professional development

Career pathways for DSNs along with many other clinical nurse specialists were non-existent until the development of nurse consultant posts (Walters 2000). This gave them a direction of career travel instead of the glass ceilings many were facing. There had been no agreed or implemented definition of specialist practice by the profession's regulatory body the United Kingdom Central Council (UKCC) for Nursing and Midwifery prior to its demise. Job descriptions varied across the UK in terms of essential and desirable qualities of post holders: ranging from diplomas to degrees, and teaching and diabetes course qualifications. Grading, pay and responsibilities also varied enormously (Da Costa 2000). Since coming into post, I have attained two diabetes courses, a further education teaching certificate, a B.Sc. in professional practice and I am currently taking a Masters level course in business administration. Most of my DSN colleagues have diplomas or degrees and diabetes courses. Our nursing team attends national and regional meetings to keep up to date with new technologies and developments in diabetes care and to develop their practice.

DSNs work within diabetes teams, consisting of medical colleagues (diabetologists, specialist registrars), podiatrists, dieticians and administrative staff. We all run clinics within the diabetes centre, sometimes all together, which means we can ask each others' opinion when required. How do I know that I am and remain competent to run these clinics? Through ongoing formal and informal education and updating, through working within my scope of professional practice and through working as an expert practitioner. I am not afraid to ask colleagues for help, who are always happy to offer this. When new DSNs have joined our team, we have all mentored them, supervised their initial clinics with them and remained a resource thereafter. We do not have a formal process of clinical supervision and our hospital does not have a policy on this. One of the successes is that we work in an atmosphere of mutual respect, which one might term informal clinical supervision. This means that questions are welcomed, advice is given and no one is protective about the patients they see. We see the benefits of this mutual collaboration on a daily basis.

Neither do we have identified competencies. Analysis of any formal competency structure reveals a very loose system, but I believe my colleagues and I are competent. I believe this through informal means: what they ask me about and the gaps they find in their knowledge. We have created a culture of supporting each other through shared learning and that it is OK to ask, rather than risk causing patient harm through ignorance. This operationalises the *Scope of Professional Practice* (UKCC 1992). If mistakes were to happen, we believe it is an opportunity to reflect and learn, rather than to punish.

In January 2002, I became a Nurse Consultant within the department. The primary role change included leadership, research, audit, service design and consultancy. This role gives me the legitimacy to work across our Trust, Primary Care Trust (PCT) and across professions. This enables service development and redesign and a chance to impact upon organisational change and nursing strategy, which differs from my role as a DSN.

I am confident I am working at an advanced level because this was the point at which the national nurse consultant functions were based (NHS Executive 1999). These included an expert practice function, together with those in professional leadership and consultancy and education, training and development. Despite what may be termed the limitations in the process of assessment, these core functions were discussed verbally at interview and importantly have enabled ongoing personal reflection in the light of my previous knowledge and skills.

I would also consider some of my DSN colleagues who are not nurse consultants to be working at an advanced level in clinical practice. In addition, the nurse consultant competencies may offer a way of determining these for DSNs. I do support competency based role development as it makes it clearer what the next step could be and highlights what skills and what resources are needed. It certainly appears a great omission from our current practice, even at the basic level of defining the roles that we undertake.

Over the last few years we have developed specialist nurse-led clinics, in antenatal care, paediatrics, teenage and young adult groups. Each clinic has a nurse specifically trained in diabetes and in the needs of the client group. A paediatric-trained DSN nurses the under 14–16 age group and links with an adult-trained DSN who works with the paediatric team to manage the teenagers' care. This is notably their transfer from the paediatric to her own teenage clinic, before ultimately joining the young adult clinic. We also have a specialist diabetes midwife, who manages the nursing expertise in the ante- and post-natal clinics and pre-conceptual care. Our aim in these nurse-led clinics is to provide a seamless transfer of care, with specialist input, throughout our patients' journey. This is particularly important for teenage diabetics, because many are lost to diabetes care when they leave the paediatric service. Therefore managing the transition clinic is very important.

In 1998, the United Kingdom Prospective Diabetes Study Group (UKPDS 33 1998; UKPDS 38 1998) recommended the early transfer to insulin treatment for type 2 patients if hyperglycaemia persisted. We recognised that the numbers of our patients requiring such treatment was increasing and due to static resources, their waiting times for what we term 'insulin transfer' were also increasing. This led to an innovative solution, with nurse-led group insulin transfer clinics, which became a research study from January 2003. The DSN who is overall lead for these sessions has developed a process whereby biomedical and quality of life measurements are taken via questionnaire at the start and at the end of the four-session programme, which lasts for approximately 12 weeks. We feel it is as important to assess the patients' perceptions of the treatment as well as biomedical indicators of improvement on insulin treatment, that is reduced blood glucose and the results of a HbA1c test*.

Patients attend with their partners and form a group for a four-session programme, where they are given a choice of insulin pens. Insulin pens are preferred to syringes and vials because they are generally easier to use. They are the size of a chunky cartridge pen and are therefore easier to handle. Insulin doses are dialled up prior to each injection using an easily viewed display and are both discreet and portable. The patient and the DSN select insulin regimes which reflect the patient's lifestyle. Support in dietary issues is provided with the dietitian. This is accompanied by teaching the ability to self manage and adjust insulin doses according to lifestyle demands and changes. The research results will be both interesting and useful to future planning and the development of nurse-led clinics. The details of these sessions are in Box 8.2.

Once again, DSNs involved in these sessions have substantial experience in teaching groups of patients and their partners who have varied diabetic needs. The DSNs consequently transfer these skills to their regular teaching on our diploma and degree programmes in diabetes, created in conjunction with our local university. These programmes form part of the modular Diploma in Professional Practice and the B.Sc. in Professional Practice, validated by the University of Brighton. Education, through sharing professional knowledge and expertise, is one of the core competencies of both nurse consultants and DSNs. An education, training and development function is identified in the health service circular

---

*HbA1c is a blood test which measures the stability and level of blood glucose retrospectively over a two- to three-month period. This gives a good overall picture of control, rather than a snapshot of blood glucose at a point in time (Audit Commission 2000: 119).

---

**Box 8.2    Insulin transfer programme**

- Once referred using our insulin transfer audit form, patients are invited to a pre-insulin transfer session with the DSN and dietitian. This aims to update patient's and partner's knowledge about diabetes, treatments, complications and risk factors. It includes the benefits of insulin treatment, the process of transferring to insulin and dietary advice.
- Two to three weeks later the patient attends the insulin transfer session. A practical demonstration of the injection technique is provided, assembling pen devices and storage.
- Preventing and managing hypoglycaemic occurrences, contacting the Driver and Vehicle Licensing Centre (DVLC)* and answering any questions or concerns.
- Four weeks later – a session on dietary management.
- Eight weeks later – a reflection on experiences with insulin, in addition to advice regarding travelling and illness, and learning to make personal adjustments to the drug dose.
- Patients can contact DSNs directly via the telephone for advice and support between these sessions.

---

regarding nurse, midwife and health visitor consultants (NHS Executive 1999). We regard this as equally important for the DSN post. The DSNs and myself as module leader, have developed and marketed these courses, which are positively evaluated and are always oversubscribed. These courses are currently learning outcome based and all DSNs have attended these and other diploma or degree modules. At each individual performance review (IPR) learning needs are identified and planning within the DSN team allows for study leave. Our philosophy is that learning by team members must be shared and must develop colleagues, as well as the individual.

However, it must be highlighted here that the courses attended by DSNs and which aim to ensure competence within new nursing and technological developments, have been initiated by the nursing and diabetes team and not through national guidance or directives. These clinics could still be run by DSNs who have not received such education and updating. It remains the personal responsibility of the DSNs to behave professionally and to protect the public by staying within their scope of practice. There is no governing body currently assessing fitness for and boundaries of practice, although this may ultimately change (see future trends in nurse-led clinics).

---

*If you have diabetes treated with insulin or tablets, by law, you must inform the DVLC.

## Measuring clinical effectiveness

Having set up DSN-led clinics, it is important to evaluate whether our resources are wisely invested. Direct feedback from patients regarding the nurse-led clinics, has been positive in terms of the benefits of time spent, lifestyle negotiations and the depth of knowledge utilised by the nursing staff. One must acknowledge, however, the bias to be favourable in a patient who wishes to continue to use a service they are evaluating. In comparison with medical clinics, the nurse-led clinics have lower non-attendance rates which suggests patients want to attend.

The advice given regarding what to do when a patient becomes ill, including continuing to give insulin and monitor blood glucose, we know keeps patients out of hospital, as it prevents rising blood glucose leading to diabetic emergencies, such as keto-acidosis. Such admissions to our intensive care are now rare, as are patients attending our Accident and Emergency Department requiring such treatment. Patient feedback also informs us that this advice is taken and they reduce their blood glucose and remain at home.

It could be argued that we do not know that the service we provide is in the patient's best interest, because we do not ask that question. However, given the range of interventions we support our patients with, we are aware that we should do more audits or research and act upon their outcomes. The difficulty is that patient referrals, expectations and the complexities of treatment are increasing, unlike staffing numbers and there is the usual dilemma of reactive dominating proactive care. By this I mean that we can become so focussed on seeing patients and therefore reacting to demands, that we do not step back and consider whether our current processes are the best way of delivering care and whether anticipating needs, rather than reacting to them, would provide better care for our patients. Reactive rather than proactive care is also emphasised by waiting lists, which are a huge political issue and patient access and reducing these lists therefore remain top of our organisational agenda. This puts diabetes services under great pressure regarding demand (which we know is increasing) and priorities. It feels as if we are so busy providing the service, that there is little time for anything else.

However, looking outside of diabetes, there are studies that suggest that the outcomes of nurse-led clinical interventions are more effective than those that are traditionally medically-led interventions (Day *et al.* 1992). This is together with approaches regarding how specialist nurses could successfully manage specific interventions (Willoughby and Burroughs 2001), client groups (Mathias *et al.* 1998) or those with gestational diabetes (Pullen *et al.* 1998). Although further research into nurse-led clinics is needed, the findings from these studies suggest they could also be relevant to diabetes nursing.

## Future trends in nurse-led clinics

Both the Audit Commission (2000) and the NSF standards (DOH 2001) suggest that specialist care will become more involved in supporting diabetes care in the community, through education and direct care. The latter may involve DSN clinics taking place in GP practices offering specialist nursing advice to patients within their own practices, and at the same time, being a clinical resource, whilst educating practice nurses and GPs. Our current nurse-led clinics could easily move, as they are not dependent on technology, other than patients being registered at some point on our database. The only consideration would be where the consultation was documented, in hospital or GP notes. A potential way forward could be patient-held notes, which are being piloted around the UK and is a project our team is currently investigating.

I believe that there would be many benefits in moving nurse-led clinics out into the community, as long as they are sufficiently resourced and do not disadvantage any other patient group, such as hospital inpatients.

The Royal Colleges (of Nursing, Physicians and General Practitioners) and Diabetes UK (a national charity supporting people with diabetes) have been collaborating to develop a performance framework for self-assessment and external peer review of diabetes services. Pilot site assessment notes and diabetes care objectives have been developed and in collaboration with Innove (formerly the Centre for Health Care Development) a web-based service assessment tool (DiabetesE), for use by PCTs and healthcare professionals is available. Further information can be obtained through e-mail from diabetes@innove.info. This may well impact upon nurse-led clinics and other structures and processes currently used in diabetes care.

On a local level, we as a DSN team will need to evaluate whether our service reflects our patients' needs and be prepared to continually assess and innovate to use our scant resources wisely. Chapter One discussed involving patients' views in service development. We are continually achieving this by using information from patient focus groups to design and adapt services, such as our nurse-led clinics and the practice environment itself. Examples include extending the times for telephone access to DSNs as this was valued highly by patients, providing a light and airy waiting area in the diabetes centre and having a specific room for patient education within the diabetes centre. The major cost in diabetes care is personnel and like many other teams, we are under-resourced for our local population. We should have six full time DSNs, whereas we only have four full time equivalents. Four are part time and only two are full time. Therefore, any additional nurse-led clinics can only be commenced if we stop doing something else, which not only raises ethical dilemmas, but may only shift, rather than solve, a problem.

## Conclusions

Nurse-led clinics in diabetes have arisen due to an innovative response by nurses to meet the increasing demand by patients for their nursing skills. National guidelines, along with standards of training required to run such clinics, have been absent. Clarification about what constitutes specialist practice has not been formally provided by regulatory bodies (see Chapter One). It remains the responsibility of individual nurses to work within their scope of professional practice, to keep updated because healthcare is dynamic, and to ensure that they have the appropriate skills to enable their patients to self care and to reduce the risk of acute and chronic complications. It is also important to respect the patient in following the path in life they choose.

Whilst questionnaire data from patients with diabetes evaluate such clinics positively, there is little direct research to demonstrate that they improve patient outcomes. The research already discussed could indeed be applied to nurse-led clinics in diabetes, but more research is obviously needed, as there is currently little evidence on the general and cost effectiveness of the processes used to provide diabetes care in either primary or specialist care (Audit Commission 2000: 101). What is important is that care is provided by enthusiastic, well-informed professionals (Audit Commission 2000: 101). Having the knowledge is obviously important, but it is not enough. It is wanting to and being able to make a difference to our patients' lives that is the key. That is and always has been the philosophy of our nurse-led clinics.

## References

Audit Commission (2000) *Testing Times. A review of diabetes services in England and Wales*, London: Audit Commission.

Bliss, M. (2000) *The Discovery of Insulin*, 3rd edn, Toronto: University of Toronto Press.

British Diabetic Association (1995) *Diabetes in the UK 1996*, British Diabetic Association.

British Medical Association (2002) *The Future Healthcare Workforce. Discussion Paper 9: A Future Model for the Healthcare Workforce*, London: BMA.

Da Costa, S. (2000) 'Diabetes Specialist Nursing: looking to the future, learning from the past', Focus on specialist nursing (Supplement), *British Journal of Nursing* 9(5), 287–290.

Day, J.L., Metcalfe, J. and Johnson, P. (1992) 'Benefits provided by an integrated education and clinical diabetes centre: a follow-up study', *Diabetic Medicine* 9(9), 855–859.

DCCT (1993) 'The effect of intensive treatment of diabetes on the development and progression of long-term complications in insulin-dependent diabetes mellitus. The Diabetes Control and Complications Trial Research Group', *New England Journal of Medicine* 329, 977–986.

Department of Health (2001) *National Service Framework for Diabetes: Standards*, London: DOH.

Mathias, M., While, A. and Shah, S. (1998) 'Nurse-led diabetes clinics benefit black and Asian patients', *Nursing Times* 94(45), 54–55.

NHS Executive (1999) *HSC 1999/217, Nurse, Midwife and Health Visitor Consultants: Establishing Posts and Making Appointments*, London: NHSE.

Pullen, F., Thompson, T. and Drubra, U. (1998) 'A nurse-led clinic for women with IGT following gestational diabetes', *Journal of Diabetes Nursing* 2(4), 115–119.

UKCC (1992) *Scope of Professional Practice*, London: United Kingdom Central Council (available through the Nursing and Midwifery Council, London).

UKPDS 33 (1998) 'Intensive blood-glucose control with sulphonylureas or insulin compared with conventional treatment and risk of complications in patients with type 2 diabetes', *Lancet* 352, 837–853.

UKPDS 38 (1998) 'Tight blood pressure control and the risk of macrovascular and microvascular complications in type 2 diabetes', *British Medical Journal* 317, 703–713.

University of York (1999) 'Complications of diabetes: screening for retinopathy, management of foot ulcers', *NHS Centre for Reviews and Dissemination* 5(4), 1–12.

Viberti, G.C., Marshall, S., Beech, R. *et al.* (1996) 'Report on Renal Disease in Diabetes', *Diabetic Medicine* 13(Suppl 4), S6–S12.

Walters, G. (2000) 'Managing new roles within the service', in Humphris, D. and Masterson, A. (eds) *Developing New Clinical Roles. A Guide for Health Professionals*, Edinburgh: Churchill Livingstone, pp. 98–121.

White, P. (2000) 'Let's celebrate the difference between doctors and nurses' (letter), *British Medical Journal* 321, 698.

Williams, G. and Pickup, J.C. (1999) *Handbook of Diabetes*, 2nd edn, Oxford: Blackwell Science.

Willoughby, D. and Burroughs, D. (2001) 'A CNS managed diabetes foot-care clinic; a descriptive survey of characteristics and foot-care behaviours of the patient population', *Clinical Nurse Specialist* 15(2), 52–57.

Yudkin, J.S., Blauth, C., Drury, P. *et al.* (1996) 'Prevention and management of cardiovascular disease in patients with diabetes mellitus: an evidence base', *Diabetic Medicine* 13(Suppl 4), S101–S121.

# Index

Note: Boxes are indicated by **bold page numbers**, Figures and Tables by *italic page numbers*, and footnotes by suffix 'n'

eBooks – at www.eBookstore.tandf.co.uk

# A library at your fingertips!

eBooks are electronic versions of printed books. You can store them on your PC/laptop or browse them online.

They have advantages for anyone needing rapid access to a wide variety of published, copyright information.

eBooks can help your research by enabling you to bookmark chapters, annotate text and use instant searches to find specific words or phrases. Several eBook files would fit on even a small laptop or PDA.

**NEW:** Save money by eSubscribing: cheap, online access to any eBook for as long as you need it.

## Annual subscription packages

We now offer special low-cost bulk subscriptions to packages of eBooks in certain subject areas. These are available to libraries or to individuals.

For more information please contact webmaster.ebooks@tandf.co.uk

We're continually developing the eBook concept, so keep up to date by visiting the website.

# www.eBookstore.tandf.co.uk